The LOGIC *of* HEALTH-CARE REFORM

THE GRAND ROUNDS PRESS

The LOGIC *of* HEALTH-CARE REFORM

PAUL STARR

WHITTLE DIRECT BOOKS

THE GRAND ROUNDS PRESS

The Grand Rounds Press presents original short books by distinguished authors on subjects of importance to the medical profession.

The series is edited and published by Whittle Books, a business unit of Whittle Communications L.P. A new book is published approximately every three months. The series reflects a broad spectrum of responsible opinions. In each book the opinions expressed are those of the author, not the publisher or advertiser.

I welcome your comments on this unique endeavor.

William S. Rukeyser
Editor in Chief

To Rebecca, Olivia, Raphael, and Abigail

Photographs: Harris Wofford: Todd Buchanan/Black Star, page 12; Alain Enthoven: Courtesy of Stanford
University News and Publications Services, page 49; John Garamendi: AP/Wide World Photos, page 63.

Charts: Linda Eckstein. Sources: *Health Affairs*, Summer 1990 and Fall 1991 (data from Harvard-Harris-ITF
1990 Ten-Nation Survey, and OECD Health Data, 1991), page 18; "EBRI Special Report and Issue Brief
Number 123," February 1992 (data from Current Population Survey , March 1991), page 20; Alliance for
Health Reform, "Health Care in America," May 1992 (based on "EBRI Issue Brief," February 1991), page
23; HCFA, National Center for Education Statistics, and *Statistical Abstract of the United States*, 19th edition,
page 24; *Health Affairs*, Fall 1991 (based on *OECD Health Systems Facts and Trends* and OECD Health Data,
1991), page 27; *Medical Economics*, November 4, 1991, page 28; AMA's *Physician Characteristics in the U.S.,
1992*, page 37; U.S. Congressional Budget Office (based on data from *Health Affairs*, Winter 1991), page 41;
Paul Starr, page 48; U.S. General Accounting Office report, "Private Health Insurance: Problems Caused by
a Segmented Market," July 1991, page 54; California Insurance Commissioner's report, "California Health
Care in the 21st Century," page 64.

The Grand Rounds Press: Martha Hume, Senior Editor; Ken Smith, Design Director;
Hillari Dowdle, Associate Editor; Susan Brill, Associate Art Director

Library of Congress Catalog Card Number: 92-85362
Starr, Paul
The Logic of Health-Care Reform
ISBN 1-879736-09-8
ISSN 1053-6620

Acknowledgments

Writing requires cooperation, tolerance, and forgiveness, especially if the writer has a large family and diligent editors. I am indebted not only to them but to a number of people who took the time (when there wasn't much) to give me comments on the original manuscript even though they may have disagreed in significant respects. I would like to thank Linda Bergthold, Alain Enthoven, Alan Hillman, Jon Kingsdale, Theodore R. Marmor, Jeremy Rosner, Steven Schroeder, Harold Stein, and Walter Zelman. I regret that I could not take all their suggestions, although I reserve that right for future projects. This book also reflects the many ideas of my wife, Sandra, who helped think about the book before a word was written.

CONTENTS

PREFACE 11

CHAPTER ONE
A Negative Consensus 16

CHAPTER TWO
What Went Wrong? 25

CHAPTER THREE
Hope Amid the Ruins 33

CHAPTER FOUR
The Logic of Systemic Reform 43

CHAPTER FIVE
Breaking the Employer Linkage 52

CHAPTER SIX
Budget Globally, Choose Locally 62

CHAPTER SEVEN
From Here to Reform 76

PREFACE

One evening in early October 1991, I sat in a living room in a suburb of Philadelphia talking about health insurance with Harris Wofford, whose name I had first heard only a few months before when he was appointed to the Senate on the death of John Heinz. Now running against former U.S. attorney general Richard Thornburgh for the rest of Heinz's term, Wofford was fighting his way up from a 40-point deficit in early polls. A few days earlier, his campaign manager, James Carville, had read an article of mine on the growing anxieties of the middle class about health insurance and called me to say Wofford agreed with my analysis. Could I come down from Princeton to help the senator work through the issue? He had been making national health insurance the centerpiece of his campaign, and by that October evening, with 33 days to go, the polls put him only 12 points behind.

Not everyone that fall thought campaigning on health insurance was a smart choice. E. J. Dionne of *The Washington Post* called health care "the issue from hell"—too complex and too costly to catch fire with the voters. One of the best-informed researchers on public opinion and health care, Robert Blendon of the Harvard School of Public Health, told a reporter that health care was a "third-tier" issue—way behind the economy, drugs, abortion, the budget deficit, and the savings and loan fiasco. Many once-ardent advocates of national health insurance had given up hope and either had quit trying to pass a program or were backing incremental changes. In the White House, President Bush was ignoring the issue.

But some analysts and politicians held a different view of the depth of discontent and the possibilities for comprehensive reform.

For years supporters of universal health insurance had framed it as an ethical challenge to help others in need; the problem, as they saw it, was how to spread to the poor one of the blessings enjoyed by the middle class. By the end of the 1980s, the issue had fundamentally changed. As health costs soared, businesses began to regard health benefits as an unmanageable burden; employers cut back benefits, insurance companies added preexisting-condition exclusions and sought to screen out high-risk subscribers, and many in the middle class found that they had insecure protection. In their eyes health insurance had changed from a problem that affects "them" to one that affects "us." That not only widened the potential constituency for reform; it also converted health insurance from a poverty issue into a general problem of economic security. Wofford's upset landslide victory in Pennsylvania telegraphed the significance of that change to the country.

Yet three daunting obstacles stand in the way of action. The health-care problem is genuinely complex; ideological conflict blocks any clear understanding; and the best-organized interests in health care benefit from the present system because of the simplest equation of medical economics: *The costs of health care equal incomes from health care.* Rising costs have meant rising incomes; controlling costs means controlling incomes. The health-care industry now represents more than one-eighth of the U.S. economy, and the stakeholders in that industry—not just physicians, but hospitals, makers of medical equipment and pharmaceuticals, venture capitalists, and insurance companies—are not about to sit out a political battle that could so greatly affect their interests, and in some cases their survival.

Earlier efforts to pass universal health insurance faced obstacles that in some ways were less daunting. National health insurance programs were introduced in Europe, Canada, and elsewhere when health care was a relatively minor industry and often before health insurance had a chance to develop commercially. Governments bought off doctors by increasing their incomes. Indeed, despite their prior opposition, American doctors profited from the introduction of Medicare in 1965. Most likely they would also have gained, at least in the short term, from health-insurance programs proposed in three earlier periods—before World War I, during the New Deal, and under the Truman administration. On sending his national health plan to Congress in 1945, President Truman noted that medical services "absorb only about 4 percent of the national income," and he declared, "We can afford to spend more for

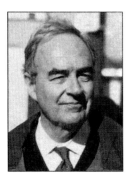

Harris Wofford's 1991 win in the race to succeed Pennsylvania senator John Heinz alerted politicians to the seriousness of voter concern about health care.

health." We could—and, in the years that followed, we did.

Sweetening the medicine of reform by paying doctors and hospitals more is no longer a political option. The imperatives have now changed, and universal access to health insurance is only part of what we need. The other part involves a fundamental reorganization of health-care finance to ensure that costs grow at a controllable rate. Indeed, I favor universal health insurance not as a way to spend more money on health care but because, properly designed, universal insurance offers the best chance and fairest method of curbing growth in the future, as it has done in the rest of the industrialized world.

Thus my view of the problem is almost exactly the opposite of the conventional view. Most Americans wonder why we have not controlled health spending and how much more national health insurance might cost. I believe that we have not controlled costs because we lack the financial control that a comprehensive health-insurance program produces.

Interest-based opposition to cost control may be enough, at least in the short run, to defeat any comprehensive health-care reform. Ideological opposition makes the challenge even more formidable. From the earliest conflicts over government health-insurance programs the issue has evoked much sharper ideological differences in the United States than in Europe. European conservatives not only supported but often introduced national health insurance programs that American conservatives denounced as socialized medicine.

The debate in the United States has had a more inflammatory character, as opponents of publicly sponsored health insurance have typically sought to identify it with alien and subversive forces. The proposal died first in 1918, when it was labeled an insidious German idea. It died a second time in the 1930s and '40s under a cloud of charges that the notion was Soviet-inspired. Lately conservatives have condemned Canada's national health insurance as an alien socialist scheme that individualistic Americans would never accept—even though Canada's health-care providers are private and Canadians choose freely among them.

The much denounced threat of national health insurance to free choice is an old canard, one that is especially misleading today. The reality is that Americans are losing freedoms under the present system. Many people fear to change jobs because they would lose coverage of an existing health condition. That is a genuine loss of economic liberty. Many have been channeled by their employers into health plans that no longer allow them to go to their personal physicians. And for the millions without insurance of any kind, "free choice" is a cruel way to describe their dependence on emergency rooms and exclusion from routine access to care. Universal coverage is itself a choice-expanding policy, and a good universal health insurance program can be designed specifically for American circumstances, to increase the real options we have.

Moreover, physicians, like consumers, have been losing freedom under the present system. The very failure to control costs in the United States has led both business and government to impose more extensive microregulation on health care than exists in countries with national health insurance. Many physicians from Europe, even from Great Britain, have commented that American doctors now face more paperwork, more regulations, more second-guessing of their decisions than is customary in countries where the government sets overall budgetary limits but leaves the detailed decisions about health care to the professionals.

And as costs grow and insurance deteriorates, American doctors see more patients who cannot afford proper care and are postponing treatment of a health problem for fear of the expense. Increasingly, doctors feel the health-insurance system interferes with the practice of good medicine. So, instead of insisting that no reform in health-care finance is needed, many in the medical profession have added their voices to those arguing on behalf of change—even fundamental change.

The approach to reform I take here attempts to enhance the liberty of consumers and providers and to meet the other great challenges of health policy: to secure equitable health coverage for all Americans, control of costs, high quality of care, and innovation.

The basic idea is not complicated: a public framework for insurance that allows Americans to choose among a variety of private health plans. But in America's highly polarized health-care debate, the concept of a national health insurance program with competing private plans is exceptionally difficult to communicate. People immediately try to classify it on one side or the other of the ideological divide. If they hear "national" first, they identify it with a total government takeover. If they hear "competition" first, they identify it with the market approaches that reject the very idea of a common responsibility to assure universal health coverage. Oversimplified media reports rarely get the idea straight.

The confusion has been aggravated by a mix-up of the terms *managed care* and *managed competition*. Managed care describes a type—actually, several types—of health-insurance plan. Managed competition refers to an approach to regulating the competition among plans, not all of which are based on managed care. Properly designed, managed competition would inhibit the growth of some managed-care plans that now flourish only because they enroll healthy beneficiaries.

To add further to the confusion, managed competition refers to a way of organizing choices under both employment-based and publicly financed insurance programs. Some reports and editorials have specifically counterposed managed competition and national health insurance, as if the two were mutually exclusive. Yet in 1977, when Stanford economist Alain Enthoven first outlined a proposal for managed competition, it was presented and understood as an option for national health insurance.

In recent years the phrase *national health insurance* has increasingly become identified with a federally financed and regulated insurance system—a more narrow conception than was current only a decade ago. When I use the words national health insurance, I mean a system that provides access to a mainstream standard of coverage on the basis of citizenship rather than employment. All Americans would be included, and residents who are not citizens could qualify for coverage through their own or a family member's legal employment or study.

No proposal for health-care reform can satisfy all the interests in health care, much less overcome the ideological divisions that exist between different groups and even within the medical profession. My aim is to cut through some of the fog that envelops the issue and foster a clearer understanding of the alternatives open to us today. National health policy is not a riddle without an answer. Unless we are ready to give up on the idea of self-government, surely we can do at least as well in providing universal coverage, controlling costs, and satisfying public demands as the other capitalist democracies of the West.

CHAPTER ONE

A NEGATIVE CONSENSUS

I t was a crisis. So said the news media. So said three-quarters of the public, according to surveys. So said the political leaders of both parties. All agreed that Americans faced a health-care crisis created by "skyrocketing" costs, rampant inefficiency, and the continued lack of insurance coverage for millions of people. Seizing on the issue, Democrats in Congress called for national health insurance. On the defensive, a Republican president concerned about reelection proposed an alternative that relied more on the private sector.

The year was 1971. A Rip Van Winkle who fell asleep then and awoke 20 years later would have rubbed his eyes at a world transformed. Communism had collapsed in Eastern Europe, Germany had reunited, and the Soviet Union had disappeared from the map. But at least one thing would have been familiar. Americans were still fighting the same political battles over health care. The media were abuzz with talk of a health crisis, Democrats were proposing national health insurance, and a Republican president concerned about reelection was touting a market-oriented alternative.

Yet if our Rip Van Winkle began to ask what had happened over the two previous decades, he would soon find that the realities of health care had changed profoundly. Consider the following:

Since 1970 the economic stakes in the battle over health care have risen sharply. In 1970 *Business Week* called health care a "$60 billion crisis"; by 1991 the cost was approaching—and now exceeds—$800 billion a year. Health-care spending had risen from 7.3 percent to 13.2 percent of GNP. Since 1980, health care has consumed an additional 1 percent of GNP *every 35 months.*

The trend of expanding health-insurance coverage has been reversed. In the three decades before 1970 employer-based health plans and public programs covered an increasing proportion of Americans. But in the 1980s coverage stopped growing and the ranks of the uninsured began to expand.

Conventional health insurance is giving way to alternatives that often restrict consumers' choice of physicians and regulate physicians' choices of treatment. In 1970 most Americans had health-insurance plans that reimbursed them for fee-for-service charges by whatever doctors and hospitals they chose and for virtually all recommended tests and treatments. By 1990 health maintenance organizations (HMOs) and other forms of managed care were becoming dominant, imposing restrictions that many doctors and patients would not have accepted two decades ago.

The health-care industry has undergone other fundamental changes over the past two decades. The doctor shortage of the 1970s has turned into a glut in the 1990s—at least of specialists, who have poured onto the market in record numbers (even though in some communities primary-care physicians continue to be relatively scarce). New types of ambulatory health centers and home health-care businesses have proliferated, and many such services, as well as hospitals, are now owned and run by national chains. The provision of health care has changed in character from a traditional, low-key professional ethos to a more entrepreneurial, marketing orientation, aimed in part at stimulating new demands. Whole new medical technologies have arrived, the fruit of decades of biomedical research and an emerging revolution in biotechnology.

In a sense, the glut of specialists, the turn toward health-care marketing, and the advent of new technologies are the fulfillment of policies adopted decades ago to spur medical research and education and the expansion of facilities. These policies have indeed produced some of the benefits originally hoped for. But from the standpoint of cost containment, they are like a time bomb detonating years after being planted, setting off serial explosions and side effects that no one foresaw.

Why Americans Want Change

Discontent with America's health-care system is almost palpable. Polls now regularly find that 90 percent of Americans believe either that fundamental change is needed in health care or that the entire system has to be rebuilt. Employers are equally unhappy. A

High spending, high dissatisfaction

Costs vs. public reactions to the health-care systems in five countries

Per capita spending (U.S. dollars, 1989)

U.S.	
CANADA	
GERMANY	
ITALY	
BRITAIN	

0    $500 $1,000 $1,500 $2,000 $2,500

% of public dissatisfied

U.S.	
CANADA	
GERMANY	
ITALY	
BRITAIN	

0   20%   40%   60%   80%   100%

SOURCES: HARVARD-HARRIS-ITF TEN-NATION SURVEY, 1990; OECD

Among advanced societies, the U.S. ranks highest in both spending and dissatisfaction. People were "dissatisfied" if they said their system needs either "fundamental change" or to be "completely rebuilt."

1990 survey of chief executive officers at Fortune 500 companies (conducted by Gallup for the Robert Wood Johnson Foundation) found that 91 percent say the system needs fundamental change or a complete rebuilding. These views amount to a negative consensus on the American health-care system. Even the editor of *The Journal of the American Medical Association*, George D. Lundberg, declared in 1991 that fundamental reform had an air of "inevitability" about it. To many the health-care system resembles a city built on a geological fault, waiting for an earthquake.

America's troubles with health care stand out sharply in international comparisons. A study that compared public opinion about health care in 10 countries, conducted by Louis Harris and Associates in 1988 and 1990, found that the U.S., along with Italy, had the highest level of public dissatisfaction with its health-care system. Interestingly enough, public satisfaction in the countries surveyed is related to spending per capita: with lower spending generally comes higher dissatisfaction. The Italians' high dissatisfaction, for example, reflects their country's low per capita expenditures on health care. The exception is the United States, which manages to have the lowest public approval while spending more for health care than any other country (see chart, above).

The exceptional pattern of health-care spending in the United States is striking. While America is the one advanced industrialized country without national health insurance, countries with national health insurance spend less. In 1990 (the latest year for which international data are available), the leading nations in Europe and North America, as well as Japan, spent an average of 7.5 percent of their national income on health care. America's 12.4 percent that year was by far the highest. Per capita the United States spent 40 percent more on health care than Canada, the second-highest spender, and twice as much as major European nations. Year by year the gap has been growing.

To be sure, surveys indicate that while dissatisfied with the system, about three of every four Americans are satisfied with the quality of medical care they personally receive. Technically, American medicine is superb. What troubles the public, studies suggest, is the lack of secure insurance protection and uncontrolled costs.

The usual measure of the insurance problem is the number of people who are without coverage at any one time—an estimated 36 million in 1991, up almost two million from the year before. That figure represents one of six Americans under age 65, yet it understates the problem; in addition, some 40 million more Americans are estimated to be underinsured because their policies provide little protection in the event of serious illness. And according to a 1992 Census Bureau study, more than one in four Americans (26 percent) had no health-insurance coverage at some time over 28 months between 1987 and 1989—a period, as it happened, of relatively full employment.

The rising unemployment in the recession that began in 1991 undoubtedly raised the number of uninsured over a similar period, although an exact estimate is not yet available. But perhaps the biggest effect of any recession is to make insecurity about health coverage pervasive, since those worried about losing a job typically worry about losing health insurance. The linkage of insurance to jobs often doubles the loss and compounds the anxiety of unemployment. It is the peculiar evil of the American health-insurance system that when the breadwinner of a family is thrown out of work, the entire family is threatened with loss of both secure access to health care and protection against financial devastation.

Yet the unemployed are only a minority of the uninsured. The majority of Americans without insurance are either working themselves or are members of a family with an employed adult (see chart, next page). Typically they are the working poor, but many are middle class—or at least used to be. During the 1980s, these people with jobs faced the biggest losses of coverage as employers and

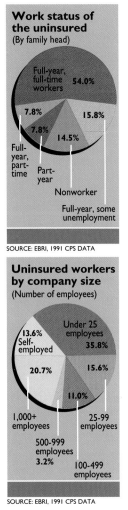

Work status of the uninsured
(By family head)

Full-year, full-time workers 54.0%

7.8%

15.8%

7.8%

14.5%

Full-year, part-time

Part-year

Nonworker

Full-year, some unemployment

SOURCE: EBRI, 1991 CPS DATA

Uninsured workers by company size
(Number of employees)

13.6% Self-employed

Under 25 employees 35.8%

20.7%

15.6%

11.0%

1,000+ employees

25-99 employees

500-999 employees 3.2%

100-499 employees

SOURCE: EBRI, 1991 CPS DATA

Nearly 36 million Americans under age 65 have no health insurance; more than 30 million of those are employed. About half of the uninsured who work are employed by companies with fewer than 100 employees.

health insurers tried to limit their own burdens and risks, often by cutting off coverage to people likely to incur high health-care costs. This is an important new trend: increasingly, Americans excluded from insurance protection are not just people with low incomes but middle-class people with above-average health risks.

The families of employees of small businesses and the self-employed have been in particular jeopardy of losing insurance (see chart, lower left). Many have faced staggering rate increases and are no longer able to afford insurance. Insurers have not only raised rates; they have "redlined" entire industries and occupations, judging them to be "uninsurable." Some of these, like florists and hair stylists, are believed to be especially likely to include HIV-positive men, while others, such as sawmill workers, are considered prone to accidents. Some insurers have even blacklisted professional groups (including physicians!) because they tend to demand a lot of health care.

Many larger employers have also structured jobs and benefit plans to keep down the number of people they insure. It is no secret how companies avoid providing health benefits. They rely on part-time or short-term workers, or they contract out work to small firms that provide no benefits. Even some local governments have discovered they can save money by contracting out to private firms with uninsured workers. Some employers have also stopped paying for coverage of dependents. As a result, the percentage of children covered by employer-sponsored insurance has dropped sharply in the past decade. And when annually renewing their contracts with employers, some insurers have begun to exclude workers or dependents who have developed high-cost conditions during the year.

This shrinkage of privately insured "risk pools" has been part of a general rollback of employer health benefits. In the face of annual premium increases averaging more than 20 percent, employers have reduced their share of premiums, added or raised deductibles and copayments, and switched to plans with more exclusions and limitations. Since 1980 the share of health premiums paid by employers has dropped from 80 percent to 69 percent. Many companies have also cut insurance coverage of their retirees as the prospect of enormous liabilities has grown.

Another step, originally taken to cut insurance costs, has also heightened employees' insecurity about health coverage. Most large employers now "self-insure," which allows them to escape state insurance regulations, including those mandating minimum levels of coverage. In 1991 a federal appeals court in New Orleans ruled in favor of a Texas company that self-insured and effectively terminated coverage of AIDS when costs for an employee suffering from the disease soared. According to the court, employers who self-insure are not legally obligated to maintain coverage. They can terminate it at any time—and some are doing just that.

In addition, some insurance companies have simply canceled coverage when policyholders have submitted large claims, or they have refused payment on the ground that the subscribers must have withheld information on the original application. And because of lax insurance regulation, says a study by the U.S. General Accounting Office, some 400,000 Americans were left uninsured between 1988 and 1990 when their insurers folded up operations. Many more workers have been stranded when their companies disappeared in bankruptcies and mergers.

Another development that adds to the public's feeling of insecurity is the growing number of health plans that exclude coverage of preexisting conditions. The majority of employers who offer insurance today have policies with such exclusions. Some plans, in fact, do not merely exclude specific conditions; they deny any coverage to individuals if they have had one of a list of serious conditions at some time in the past. Unknown 15 years ago, such clauses can have devastating effects. A child born disabled loses health coverage when a parent changes jobs. A woman whose cancer has been in remission discovers that she has no insurance coverage when another tumor is discovered after her husband has changed jobs. Under current statutes such exclusions are entirely legal.

Preexisting-condition clauses not only deny millions of Americans health coverage when they most need it; such clauses also limit opportunities for economic mobility. Many employees hesitate to change jobs now for fear of losing coverage. In a 1991 *New York Times*-CBS poll, three of 10 Americans said they or someone in their household had experienced this kind of job lock. And when people are deprived of job mobility, the economy is deprived of potentially greater contributions they could make elsewhere—an indirect and unmeasured cost of our health-care system.

Insecurity about health coverage thus involves several distinct concerns. Americans are worried not only about the risk of being uninsured; even those who are insured are worried about being denied coverage when the real need comes and of being tied down to a particular job, slaves to health insurance. The spread of exclusions and limitations, arbitrary terminations of coverage, and outright fraud are some of the reasons my Princeton colleague, economist Uwe Reinhardt, says that health insurance in America might be better called "unsurance."

Many Americans are deeply angry about being stuck with unsurance. They feel abandoned and betrayed. They worked hard for years on the assumption that they would receive certain things in return, one of them being health benefits. When they lose that protection, they see everything they have built in jeopardy.

Perhaps most disturbing, they know that all the trends in insurance coverage are moving in the wrong direction. A 1991 survey of small employers by Louis Harris found that 13 percent had recently eliminated health-insurance benefits and another 30 percent expected to be forced to drop them in the future. As health coverage evaporates, employees ask themselves how they will be able to hang on to their standard of living. Americans today do not have to be poor to worry that the system for financing health care will someday impoverish them.

Why America Needs Change

The costs and insecurities felt directly by the public are grounds enough for reform, but the health-care problem has still wider dimensions. The system's costs and indirect effects are key factors in the deeper fiscal and economic problems besetting the U.S.

The health costs that hit most Americans directly—increased employee contributions for insurance premiums and growing out-of-pocket expenses for copayments, deductibles, and uncovered services—are only the tip of the health-cost iceberg. Employees generally do not know how much their employer pays for their health insurance; few understand how large a tax subsidy they enjoy because of the exclusion of employers' contributions from taxable income. Even fewer have any idea what share of their taxes goes to health care. If anything, public perceptions are structurally biased to underestimate health-care costs. In a sense, the public dissatisfaction with health-care costs is all the more compelling because Americans have been cushioned against the full burden.

For both business and government, the rising cost of health care has become a chronic economic ailment. From 1965 to 1989, business spending on health benefits climbed from 2.2 percent to 8.3 percent of wages and salaries, and from 8.4 percent to 56.4 percent of pretax corporate profits. Some economists argue that the higher cost of health benefits has not reduced profits; they maintain—with strong supporting evidence—that the costs have come out of workers' pay instead. Most people are unlikely to find comfort in that possibility. Since the early 1970s, real take-home pay has stagnated, in part because health benefits have absorbed so large a share of increases in compensation. And despite the skepticism of professional economists, many firms are convinced that higher health-benefit costs are hurting their profitability, which is why they have reformed and cut back their benefit plans.

The impact on the public sector has been just as serious. Government costs for health care have risen 11 percent a year, three to four times above recent inflation. Because of wide resistance to higher taxes, increased health costs have necessarily cut into other public programs. In effect, health care has crowded out other needs from the public budget.

The shift of public expenditures to health care may harm not only other social needs but also economic growth. Over the past several decades, the portion of public spending devoted to investment has declined sharply. Investment in roads, bridges, and other additions to the stock of public wealth commanded 6.9 percent of public spending between 1945 and 1952 but only 1.2 percent in the 1980s. Public investments have a payoff in the future; borrowing for investment purposes has a sound economic logic. But while federal borrowing has hit record levels in the past decade, the United States has shifted public spending from investment to consumption—of which most health spending is a prime example.

The crowding out of productive public investment is one of several ways in which the growth of the health-care system now impinges on the nation's productivity. I have already mentioned the reduction of job mobility. While the insurance system locks some into jobs, it locks others into welfare. The principal alternative to welfare lies in low-paying jobs that typically do not carry health benefits. Because moving off welfare often means losing Medicaid, millions on welfare find that if they work, they cannot have secure access to health care. One major benefit of universal health insurance would be to promote the transition of the dependent from welfare to work.

In addition, health benefits have become a major source of friction between labor and management—in recent years, according to the AFL-CIO, the scaling back of health benefits has been the cause of the majority of strikes in the United States. That too is a cost of our insurance system that countries with national health insurance do not face.

Few deny that health care in America is too costly, but some are curiously indifferent to the problem. What percentage of the GNP,

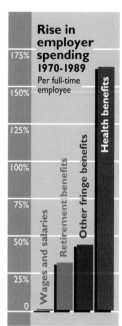

Rise in employer spending 1970-1989
Per full-time employee

Wages and salaries · Retirement benefits · Other fringe benefits · Health benefits

SOURCE: ALLIANCE FOR HEALTH REFORM, EBRI DATA

Employers' spending on health benefits has risen far more rapidly than other forms of employee compensation. Measured in constant 1989 dollars, this category grew 163 percent between 1970 and 1989.

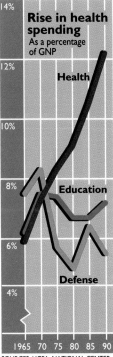

Rise in health spending
As a percentage of GNP

14%

12%
Health

10%

8%
Education

6%

Defense

4%

1965 70 75 80 85 90

SOURCES: HCFA, NATIONAL CENTER FOR EDUCATION STATISTICS, STATISTICAL ABSTRACT OF THE U.S.

The U.S. currently spends about twice as much on health care as it does on education or national defense. In the early '70s, the three sectors consumed approximately equal portions of the GNP.

they ask, is the right percentage to spend on health care? Isn't our spending for health care creating new jobs? And isn't it a natural evolutionary shift in a postindustrial service economy to spend a rising share of GNP on health care?

In the 1950s and '60s, when we were in the early stages of the health sector's expansion, these were reasonable questions. But as costs in the U.S. have risen further from the average in other advanced societies, it has become clear that a peculiar dynamic is at work in the United States, eroding real wages and the fiscal integrity of government. One comparison particularly helps to bring the rise of spending for health care into sharp relief (see chart, left). In 1965 the United States spent about the same percentage of GNP on each of three sectors—education (6.2 percent), health care (5.9 percent), and defense (7.5 percent). The military's share has now fallen beneath 6 percent and is projected to drop further during the 1990s, while education has edged up slightly to 7.2 percent. But the share spent on health care has doubled to over 13 percent in 1991. A projection by the Bush administration suggests it might reach 17 percent by the year 2000; some forecasts put it as high as 20 percent. This vast shift of national resources is proceeding without any clear understanding or public discussion of its long-term adverse repercussions for the country.

And despite this fantastic rate of spending, there is the ultimate irony: we do not have a healthier society than do Western countries that spend far less. This ought not to be surprising. Studies have long shown that spending on health care is not a major determinant of a nation's health. Yet without reform of the nation's health-care-financing system, there is no way to shift resources toward uses that would be genuinely conducive to health as well as prosperity.

Back in 1971, when our Rip Van Winkle nodded off, there was an abundance of fresh ideas about reforming the health-care system. While there was a sense of crisis, there was also optimism about possible remedies. Since then, many of those remedies have been tried without success. Now there is a readiness to go beyond mere tinkering but nowhere agreed upon to go. From the negative consensus about the status quo, Americans have not yet been able to fashion a positive consensus about an alternative. And that, in part, is because we have no clear understanding of where and why the system is failing.

CHAPTER TWO

WHAT WENT WRONG?

A mong the many explanations for America's continuing crisis of health-care costs, two lines of thought stand out. One traces rising costs to many different "cost drivers," prominently including Americans' high expectations and demands, new technologies, malpractice litigation, and the aging of the population. This approach often produces long laundry lists of recommendations for piecemeal reforms. It also encourages the perception that we are all responsible for the problems of health care and, perhaps, that no one is really responsible because high costs reflect cultural patterns and demographic trends beyond anyone's control. It is a view endorsed by much of the leadership of the health-care industry.

The second line of explanation emphasizes health-care finance and organization. While acknowledging that ingrained cultural attitudes, technological change, and aging have had some effect on costs, this approach focuses much more closely on the economic structure of the system as the key cause of America's rising costs and deteriorating insurance coverage.

I am an advocate of this systemic interpretation and, hence, of systemic reform. But before laying out that view, or at least one version of it, I want to challenge the explanations that constitute the conventional wisdom and that provide a consoling vision of the health-cost problem.

Consoling Explanation No. 1: Americans expect more. It is a comforting and even flattering thought that we have higher medical costs because Americans are especially demanding and have higher expectations than people elsewhere do. It suggests we have more sophistication and more rigorous standards than foreigners who accept "nationalized" health care. This argument implicitly warns against systemic changes that would require us to lower our expectations.

But is it true that American patients are more demanding and that these higher demands cause our higher costs? The health-care decision that is most under the control of the consumer is the initial choice to contact a doctor. If Americans really are especially demanding, we should expect them to consult physicians more frequently than people elsewhere do. Yet the annual rate of physician contacts in the United States is below average for industrialized countries. In fact, the American rate of 5.3 contacts per year is less than half that of Germany (11.5) and Japan (12.9), both of which have lower health-care costs.

This should not be surprising. The costs of the health-care systems in advanced societies are not concentrated at the front end, where consumers have most control over the care they receive. Rather, costs are concentrated later on, typically in a hospital, where doctors and health-care managers have most control over the use of resources. This pattern suggests that the incentives and constraints influencing their decisions are crucial.

The argument that Americans' high demands cause high costs assumes that high costs reflect a higher level of service. Compared with health care in other Western countries, America's system certainly does provide far more cardiac surgery and organ transplants, although less primary and preventive care. But the spending gap between the U.S. and other countries is not due primarily to the high rate of high-tech care in the U.S.

The most detailed comparisons of American with foreign health expenditures have involved Canada, which is the world's second-highest spender. Of the Canadian-U.S. expenditure difference (now amounting to about 3.5 percent of GNP), between a third and a half is due to higher administrative and insurance costs in the United States. Roughly another third reflects the higher expense of physicians' services; a carefully controlled comparison of expenditures for physicians' services in the two countries showed, however, that in 1985 and 1987 Canadians, while spending less, actually received a higher volume of physicians' services. The difference in cost was entirely explained by higher physician fees in the U.S. (The U.S. does spend more for medical research, accounting for a small percentage of the total difference in spending.)

How America stacks up internationally

	Health spending* per capita	Inpatient days per capita	Physician contacts per capita	Infant mortality per 1,000 live births	Life expectancy (male) at birth	at age 80	Percent of population age 65 and over
U.S.	$2,354	1.3	5.3	10.0	71.5	6.9	12.3%
CANADA	$1,683	2.0	6.6	7.2	73.0	6.9	11.1%
GERMANY	$1,232	3.5	11.5	7.6	71.8	6.1	15.4%
JAPAN	$1,035	4.1	12.9	4.8	75.5	6.9	11.2%
BRITAIN	$836	2.0	4.5	9.0	72.4	6.4	15.6%
OECD average for 24 nations	$1,059	2.8	6.0	10.6	72.1	6.3	13.0%

* In U.S. dollars, 1989

SOURCE: *HEALTH AFFAIRS*, FALL 1991, OECD DATA

Although the U.S. spends more for health care than any other nation, international comparisons indicate that its citizens do not necessarily receive better care than residents of nations that spend less.

Finally, the remaining gap reflects higher costs for hospital care in the United States. According to a comparative study of Canadian and American hospitals, admission rates are about the same while stays are longer in Canada. American hospital care, however, is far more costly because of what happens after admission. Costs run 50 percent greater in U.S. hospitals because the hospitals use more "inputs" (that is, they do more tests, procedures, etc.) and because the hospitals pay more for their inputs. One cause may be the much greater share of American nurses' time consumed by filling out forms required for reimbursement and regulation, which not only raises costs, but interferes with personal care.

Consumers hardly desire higher administrative and insurance costs or higher physician and hospital prices, but what about the greater intensiveness of medical care? That American medicine is more procedure-oriented and technologically intensive is a routine finding of comparative health-care research. Some analysts point to an aggressive therapeutic style evident, for example, in more radical surgical interventions favored by doctors in the United States when compared with their French and British peers. These differences in practice style seem to reflect patterns of medical training in the U.S., the much higher rate of special-

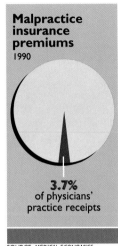

Malpractice insurance premiums
1990

3.7%
of physicians'
practice receipts

SOURCE: MEDICAL ECONOMICS,
NOVEMBER 4,1991

On average, physi-
cians pay less than
4 percent of annual
practice receipts for
malpractice insur-
ance. That amounts
to less than 1 per-
cent of total U.S.
health expenditures.

izatation among American physicians, and the financial incentives for both doctors and hospitals to emphasize procedures.

Some Americans are sufficiently well informed to expect and demand that a lot of specific tests and procedures be performed, and they might well be dissatisfied with the technology available at community hospitals in other Western countries. One study, conducted for the Robert Wood Johnson Foundation, finds that a much higher percentage of Americans than of foreigners say they would seek a second opinion if their physician said they had a terminal illness. Americans who are denied organ transplants sometimes go on radio and television to plead for public support—a phenomenon not seen elsewhere.

Still, it is hard to see how patients could have shaped the prevailing patterns of medical practice and hospital management. Most patients leave choice of treatment to their doctors. Physicians and other professionals educate the public about appropriate styles of care. In explaining differences in technological intensiveness, the direction of causality seems at least as likely to run from the health-care system to public attitudes as from public attitudes to the system.

Consoling Explanation No. 2: Malpractice litigation. Many people, especially physicians, are convinced that high malpractice-insurance rates and the practice of defensive medicine are major sources of excessive health costs in the United States. Once again, the claim is that Americans are different—more litigious as patients and more likely as jurors to give big verdicts for plaintiffs.

Yet the evidence does not bear out the hypothesis that malpractice litigation is a major source of the cost problem. Since malpractice insurance represents less than 1 percent of overall health costs, it cannot possibly be a primary cause of the growth in expenditures. To be sure, some medical specialties in some states have faced staggering rate increases. These periodic shocks reflect the cyclical nature of the insurance business and the inability of insurers to spread risks beyond the members of one specialty in one state. Overall, malpractice-insurance premiums have been virtually constant as a share of physician costs.

The impact of defensive medicine on costs is more difficult to evaluate. Although some defensive procedures are unnecessary, others represent legitimate quality assurance. There are no good estimates of the cost of the truly unnecessary procedures. We also do not know how many medical accidents and injuries defensively adopted procedures help to avoid. Thus, the *net* economic impact of defensive medicine is unclear.

Furthermore, doctors and hospitals generally make money off the procedures they perform, even if they do them defensively. Stanford health economist Victor Fuchs has asked the pointed hypothetical question: "If new legislation outlawed all future malpractice claims, by how much would physicians and hospitals voluntarily cut their present revenues?" Anyone who thinks defensive medicine is a big problem must believe that providers would sacrifice billions of dollars in revenues. This seems implausible.

Some reforms of malpractice law, such as arbitration procedures to settle cases out of court, do make sense. The tort system is not an efficient or effective way to raise the quality of care, and only a small portion of the money paid out in malpractice premiums ends up compensating plaintiffs (the great bulk being consumed by insurance companies and lawyers). Yet, as sensible as reforms may be, not even the most extensive changes in the malpractice system are likely to alter the general trend in health-care costs.

Consoling Explanation No. 3: Aging. There is no question that it costs more on average to care for the aged than for younger people and that the proportion of the aged in the population is slowly but appreciably growing. Those realities give rise to a genuine long-term problem that will be especially acute once the baby-boom generation reaches advanced old age.

But thus far aging has been only a secondary factor in overall health-sector expansion. The share of GNP devoted to health spending has not soared in recent decades because of a massive onset of old age. Moreover, age differences do not help account for international differences in health spending. The reason the U.S. spends more on health than other countries do is not that it has a larger elderly population. Among 24 industrialized nations, the U.S. ranks 17th in percentage of the population age 65 or over. In particular, the Scandinavian countries, Germany, and Britain have much larger elderly populations—about 25 percent greater relative to the U.S. As these examples illustrate, how many elderly people a country has is less important than how it manages and pays for the health care of all age groups. The U.S. system generates high costs for all Americans, and especially high costs for care of the aged, making them not the cause but a focus of the problem.

Health-care costs did rise more rapidly for the aged after the introduction of Medicare. What is more surprising is that they have continued to rise disproportionately in recent years. The remedy, however, lies less in special rules for care of the aged than in general reform of the system. Perhaps what should disturb us most is that we have already seen a vast increase in health costs before the big demographic shift toward the aged occurs in the next century.

Consoling Explanation No. 4: Technology. Those who argue that new technology is the primary cause of higher costs generally have in mind big-ticket items such as new imaging technologies, organ transplantation, intensive-care units, and renal dialysis. Such innovations have undoubtedly brought higher costs, but as we have seen, only about a third of the higher levels of U.S. spending, compared with Canada, reflects the greater expense of hospital care—and of that, only a portion is due to greater use of technology.

Certainly, there are differences in technology. For example, the U.S. has eight times more magnetic-resonance-imaging facilities than Canada on a per capita basis, and we do more than 20 times as much bypass surgery as some major European countries. But do our higher levels reflect appropriate use and sound decisions about investment? While waiting lists in Canada may reveal organizational inefficiencies and insufficient levels of investment (depending on how urgent the procedures genuinely are), many high-tech services in the United States have been overbuilt and then used for purposes for which they have never been demonstrated to be effective. For example, computerized tomography (the CT scan) radically improved treatment of head injuries, but was then misused to investigate headaches.

At the core of the problem is the relationship between doctors and hospitals. Hospitals do not sell their services directly but only through physicians, who are free to take their patients and purchasing power elsewhere. (Increasingly, physicians themselves have set up independent imaging centers and other facilities to participate directly in the profits.) To keep their beds filled, hospitals must keep their doctors happy. They duplicate costly technologies and then use them well below capacity because institutional imperatives overwhelmingly press them to do so.

In other markets, excess supply drives down prices. The supplier that refuses to cut prices loses customers and may go out of business. Why doesn't that happen in health care? The answer brings us to the heart of the matter: the perverse and peculiar features of health-care markets.

The Systemic View

The American health-care system has developed under the shaping influence of incentives for private decision-makers to expand and intensify medical services. These incentives are now entrenched in the system's physical structures and everyday practices. Their effects have been magnified by public policies that generated ever more doctors, more hospital capacity, and more technology. Then, when government and business tried to control costs, they found they had denied themselves the instruments necessary to do so.

Traditional insurance for fee-for-service medical care lacks any of the usual checks on consumption. When buying a house or a hamburger, consumers usually have to weigh the costs against other possible expenditures. They also can, and do, compare the price and value of what various sellers are offering. Under third-party health insurance, however, patients have little incentive to weigh costs carefully, and because they lack sufficient knowledge they generally rely on professionals for guidance on treatment and other critical decisions affecting costs. With some exceptions, the professionals who make the decisions increase their earnings by providing more services. It is no surprise, therefore, that many of them do so. Moreover, the fragmentation and complexity of the system generate an administrative burden of staggering dimensions.

These incentives have been built into the health-care system. They have guided investment decisions about the construction of hospitals and purchase of equipment. They have influenced young doctors' choices of specialty: we have too many surgeons and too few primary-care doctors because our financing system has for decades encouraged doctors to invest in surgical training. These incentives, moreover, have influenced the everyday rules of thumb that doctors use in deciding about tests, hospitalization, operations, and so on. American physicians' practice styles are partly the product of financial arrangements that for decades rewarded the decision to treat even if there was no good evidence the treatment would work. In short, financial incentives have become entrenched in physical assets, the distribution of specialists, and the patterns of accepted medical practice.

The result is not just incidental waste and a few flagrant abuses but a vast misallocation of resources. In the conventional fee-for-service sector, Americans experience about 960 days of hospital care per thousand persons; in prepaid group-practice plans, the comparable figure is 460 days. (The Kaiser Foundation Health Plan has even cut the number below 400.) Studies evaluating the appropriateness of care indicate that as many as 30 percent of the tests and procedures in the United States are unnecessary. Taking all the sources of inefficiency together, Arnold Relman, the former editor of *The New England Journal of Medicine*, estimates that roughly one-third of health-care expenditures are medically unnecessary.

The distortions of investment in health-care resources are not only costly; they also reduce our capacity to provide good medical care. With too many specialists but not enough primary-care physicians, we have much unnecessary surgery but too little immunization of children. With too great a supply of imaging technology, used at too low a rate, hospitals and clinics raise prices to recoup their investment, and the services become inaccessible to many who might benefit from them.

Consider the case of early detection of breast cancer through the use of mammography. With fully utilized mammography machines, a screening mammography examination should cost no more than $55, according to studies by the GAO and the Physician Payment Review Commission. But because machines are typically used far beneath capacity, prices often run double that amount. With prices so high, many women cannot afford a mammogram (indeed, at such prices, it is not clear that mammography can survive a stringent cost-benefit test). In other words, *because we have too many mammography machines, we have too little breast-cancer screening.* Only in America are poor women denied a mammogram because there is too much equipment.

This is symptomatic of the larger problem: the public-health failures of the American medical system are not the result of our spending too little; they often stem from spending too much the wrong way, thereby producing patterns of practice and organization ill-suited to primary care, prevention, and public health.

Of course, we cannot undo the past choices that have given us our present system. But we can at least begin changing the legacy that we leave to the next generation by shifting incentives away from overspecialization, overbuilding, and overspending. To do so, we need to change health-care finance systemically—that, in fact, is the great opportunity of national health reform.

HOPE AMID THE RUINS

U ncontrolled growth in costs and deepening insecurities about insurance are not only problems in health care; they are also an index of political failure. How to respond to rising health costs has been a major concern of national policy for the past 20 years, and for even longer, reformers have sought to extend insurance coverage to the entire population. Both business and government have launched countless programs attacking one or another part of the problem. There has been no shortage of research evaluating alternative approaches. But political deadlock has prevented any breakthrough.

This paralysis has created a dangerous sense of frustration and despair. Many have concluded that the problem of health spending is intractable and that there is no way to cover all of the uninsured without making things worse. Unable to control costs through minor adjustments of policy, some in Congress and state legislatures ultimately see no alternative but to adopt some system for rationing medical care (that is, consciously limiting beneficial care by administrative priorities). After all, if high expectations are responsible for our costs, we must lower them; if technological advance is responsible, we must slow it; if aging is responsible, we must set some arbitrary age limit on treatment—or so it would seem to many who hold the conventional view. Thus does a harsh realism spring from the frustrations of reform.

Yet there is, as I have suggested, an alternative view. The more than 13 percent of GNP we spend on health care should be more than enough to provide universal coverage and high quality of care.

But to achieve that goal requires a strategy for structural change to reverse the entrenched patterns of investment and behavior that will threaten the solvency of any program for universal coverage. And to figure out such a strategy, we need to understand why reform measures have failed and where, amid the ruins of policy, we can find the sources of hope and reconstruction.

The Failure of Halfway Reform

At first appearance, the best argument for believing that cost control must end in rationing is that the steps taken to control costs so far have not worked. But the reasons for that failure do not suggest that the problem is insurmountable, only that we have not addressed it coherently. While some public policies have attempted to restrain costs, others have been powerfully promoting their growth, and the most important structural forces behind the cost explosion have remained unchecked.

Early efforts to control costs, rather than altering the organization of medical practice and hospitals, created a second level of review above them. In the 1970s, the federal government and the states initiated two major regulatory efforts: utilization review, to check up on physicians' and hospitals' treatment and billing; and health-care planning agencies, to review hospitals' capital-investment decisions. Utilization-review programs retrospectively examined the paper trail of clinical decisions; consequently, reviewers were remote from the clinical scene and had no capacity to ask for new clinical data or to encourage a more cost-effective approach in particular cases. They could do nothing but deny payment afterward. The programs challenged exceptional cases of excessive cost or doubtful quality, while accepting the routine but inefficient practices that are the crux of the problem.

Similarly, the planning agencies were entirely reactive, their authority primarily negative. They advised state governments on whether or not to approve hospital expansion plans, but they had little creative, shaping power—indeed, no power at all—to limit or redirect capital investment to get better value for money. Like utilization-review programs, the health-planning agencies sought, in practice, only to curb the worst excesses of the system; they did not challenge its standard operating procedures.

Both utilization review and health planning were weak brakes applied to a vehicle being driven with the accelerator to the floor. Under fee-for-service payment, doctors profit the more services they provide. Medicare, like Blue Cross, imposed no fee schedule—

doctors were assured payment if the fees they demanded were "usual, customary, and reasonable." Cost-based reimbursement to hospitals invited the hospitals to run up costs. These were arrangements that doctors and hospitals had secured through effective lobbying. From the beginning they were a recipe for fiscal disaster.

One regulatory effort dating from the early 1970s had some modest success in restraining costs, but its limitations are also instructive. A handful of states, including Maryland, New Jersey, and New York, regulated hospital price increases and succeeded in holding down the rate of growth in hospital expenditures to a level that was somewhat beneath the national average. But hospital costs are a function of three factors: volume, price, and the intensity of services. Rate-setting slowed price increases without controlling the other sources of growth. In addition, rate-setting, like health planning, applied exclusively to hospitals. Thus it invited a shift of technology and services from hospitals into ambulatory-care centers and doctors' offices.

With the 1979 congressional defeat of federal hospital cost-containment legislation proposed by President Carter, regulatory efforts to control overall hospital costs reached a dead end, at least for a time. In the 1980s, with the advent of the Reagan administration, the emphasis in health policy was supposed to shift from regulation to competition. At the outset of the Reagan years, several models of market-oriented reform, including a bill introduced in 1978 by Representatives David Stockman and Richard Gephardt (an odd couple, in retrospect), were circulating in Washington. Among other things, pro-competitive reform called for changes in tax policy to make employees more sensitive to health-insurance costs, a broad attack on monopolistic practices in the health professions, and strong support for HMOs and other alternative health plans. But a comprehensive, pro-competitive approach to health care turned out to lack support even among Republicans, and the administration abandoned the effort. Instead, Congress enacted measures to make the federal government a more "prudent buyer" of health care and thereby limit the costs of federal programs.

The most important initiative was the new payment system that Congress adopted in 1983 to replace Medicare's previous arrangement for reimbursing hospitals. Hospitals now would be paid per admission, rather than per day and per service. Reimbursement rates, divided into some 470 diagnosis-related groups (DRGs), would be set in advance, thus putting hospitals at risk (if costs exceeded the prospective payment, it was their loss; if costs were lower, their gain). For the first time, hospitals were given a strong incentive to control costs through such measures as discharge planning.

Yet the DRG system provides no incentive to reduce unnecessary admissions, and since it affects hospitals but not doctors, it gives doctors no incentive for cost containment. Moreover, Medicare's payment system does not apply to other payers, onto which hospitals can, and do, shift costs. As a result, hospitals have continued to be profitable even at astonishingly low occupancy rates.

The federal government has also moved to reform physician payment. From its outset, Medicare reproduced and reinforced the incentives favoring "procedural" over "cognitive" services and urban over rural physicians, helping to distort the specialty and geographical distribution of physicians. The resource-based relative-value scale, the key element in the reformed payment system, ranks physician services according to the complexity of tasks and the resources they consume. Ideally, the new approach should counteract the long-standing biases in physician payment; in practice, because of concessions to specialists, its effects are likely to be modest.

These steps toward payment reform, while generally positive, have simply not been enough: they have been slow in coming, compromised in their execution, and limited in their effect because hospitals and doctors are able to shift costs to the private sector. When hospital costs are controlled, providers shift services to the ambulatory side. When the government acts to rein in costs, providers typically charge more to the privately insured. Lacking any comprehensive mechanism of control, payers have been at a sharp disadvantage in their cost-containment battles with providers.

Employers, like the federal government, have revised their health-benefit plans to limit costs. In addition to self-insuring, many have required employees to share a higher portion of costs. Cost-sharing does tend to reduce demand, but it has serious drawbacks: patients appear to cut down as much on needed as on unneeded contacts with physicians; and cost-sharing does little to reduce the costs associated with the most expensive phases of care in the hospital, where patients exercise little control. Employers adopted other measures to control these costs. Some paid for, or even required, second opinions before surgery—a measure that has had positive but limited effects. Some contracted with outside firms for case management to control the use of services, imposing requirements such as preadmission certification for hospitalization. In recent years, many companies have moved toward managed care as a comprehensive solution. Although the picture here is more complicated—and I will have more to say about it in a moment—these efforts have thus far brought little relief to employers, and no general slowing of national health expenditures.

Once facilities, technology, and manpower are in place, it is hard for any one payer, governmental or private, to do much but shift costs elsewhere. The decisions that most affect how much it costs to operate the health-care system are the "upstream" choices about what kind of system to have in the first place: investment decisions in the physical capacity of the system, its technological complexity, and the specialized training of its key decision-makers, doctors. Because of the inherent uncertainty and ambiguity of medical decisions, physicians can easily prescribe more services to fit available time and budgets. If there are more physicians, they will find more to do—more tests to run, more need of surgery, more patients requiring follow-up. Economists call this "supplier-induced demand." While the extra services provided may individually seem reasonable, they have little impact on a society's overall health.

Throughout this period of halfway regulation in the 1970s and '80s—halfway because the basic incentives for increasingly costly health services were left in place—the supply of physicians, and particularly of specialists, was rising rapidly (see chart, right). Federal policies affecting physician training adopted in the 1960s more than doubled the number of medical-school graduates, and these graduates overwhelmingly became subspecialists. Investment in hospitals and high-tech services grew rapidly, stimulated in part by generous provisions in Medicare for reimbursing hospitals' capital costs. Whatever might have been accomplished by regulation was undone by these other developments.

The regulatory programs were destined to fail because they never imposed firm ceilings on investment or expenditures, or changed the underlying incentives facing providers and patients, or required institutions to match their resources to the needs of the populations they served. In the United States, the matching of resources to the needs of populations happened in only one significant arena: health maintenance organizations. And yet here, too, reform failed to produce the general revolution in health care that business and government were seeking.

The Rise of HMOs

In the early 1970s, enthusiasm developed among politicians and health-care policymakers for home-grown organizations long described as "prepaid group practices" or "group health plans." The

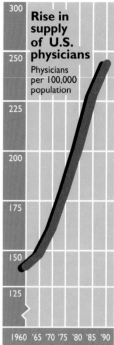

Rise in supply of U.S. physicians

Physicians per 100,000 population

300

250

225

200

175

150

125

1960 '65 '70 '75 '80 '85 '90

SOURCES: AMERICAN MEDICAL ASSOCIATION; U.S. CENSUS DATA

The number of doctors has grown far faster than the U.S. population for three decades. There are now 72 percent more physicians per 100,000 Americans than in 1960.

early group health plans, such as the Kaiser Foundation Health Plan and the Group Health Cooperative of Puget Sound, were founded in the 1930s and '40s to provide comprehensive, high-quality medical care primarily to employee groups. Almost accidentally, the plans turned out to reduce the overall costs of health care compared with conventional, fee-for-service health insurance.

Reports in the 1950s and '60s that the plans produced substantial savings set off a long and bitter debate. Many critics, especially private physicians, insisted that group health plans had lower costs only because they provided shoddy service, their enrollees were healthier, and their members were getting additional services outside the plans. Besides, they said, most Americans are too individualistic and too demanding to accept the "compromises" of a socialistic group plan. It took a lot of expensive research to show that the plans' savings were genuine, ranging from 10 to 40 percent, as compared with conventional insurance plans. The reduced costs chiefly reflected a reduced rate of hospital use. In what is generally regarded as the most reliable randomly controlled study, the Rand Corporation's health-insurance experiment in Seattle (conducted from 1976 to 1980) found savings of 28 percent from prepaid group practice with no adverse effects on health outcomes. Numerous other studies have also demonstrated that prepaid group-practice plans provide medical care of at least equal quality as fee-for-service.

Yet prepaid group practices are not easy to start. They require the development of multispecialty medical groups and special managerial skills, both of which are relatively scarce. Furthermore, as of the early 1970s, more than 30 states had laws that effectively barred prepaid group-practice plans, and most businesses did not offer them to their employees.

Searching for a distinct approach to health care, the Nixon administration in 1970 became the first to make the development of prepaid plans a central element in national health policy. The impetus came from Paul Ellwood, a Minnesota pediatric neurologist who coined the term *health maintenance organization.* (As a specialist in rehabilitation, Ellwood had become convinced that prepayment made more sense than fee-for-service.) The HMO concept included not only the prepaid group-practice plans, but also a variant, "independent practice associations" (IPAs), which were more acceptable to fee-for-service practitioners.

A peculiar feature of IPAs is that they present one face to the consumer, another to the physician. They charge capitation rates to subscribers (or their employers) but provide care through doctors in private practice, whom they generally pay by fee-for-service, although at a discount from their usual rates. (The difference is often withheld in a fund for profit-sharing at year's end.) Compared with prepaid group-practice plans, IPAs are less costly to launch, and they do not necessarily require patients to give up their family physician. However, they lack many of the organizational capacities that group-practice plans have for assuring quality and promoting conservative physician practice styles.

As HMOs have evolved over the past two decades, further varieties have emerged. Some IPAs rely on a primary-care physician to control referrals and hospitalization. These doctors are known as gatekeepers and are sometimes paid by capitation rather than by fee-for-service. While financial arrangements vary, plans that offer doctors incentives to control referrals may create a conflict between physicians' pocketbook interests and decisions about additional patient care. Such ethical dilemmas, however, are scarcely unknown in the fee-for-service sector, since a family practitioner may worry that a patient referred to a specialist may never come back.

With the inclusion of IPAs and gatekeeper plans, the original idea of prepaid group practice changed dramatically. The early organizations began with a commitment to comprehensive care and incidentally turned out to have lower costs. The new organizations were created to cut costs, but not all of them have done so in the same way. Instead of creating a distinctive organizational culture with a more conservative practice style, many of the new plans seek discounts from fee-for-service physicians and use financial incentives to reduce supplier-controlled demand. Financial incentives do affect costs, but whether these organizations are as successful as other HMOs in maintaining the quality of care is less clear.

As a result of legislation passed in 1973, the government began providing start-up grants to HMOs and requiring firms with more than 25 employees to offer at least one qualified HMO as part of an employee health plan. Congress also revised Medicare to encourage HMO enrollment among the elderly. But all of these measures have had a troubled history. The grants program ended in 1981, and Medicare's HMO provisions have failed to bring about any major shift of the elderly into prepaid plans. The requirement that employers offer a qualified HMO is still in effect, but HMOs are reluctant to force employers to comply. Yet while continuing to face enormous difficulties, HMOs have grown in number and enrollment—slowly in the East, more rapidly in the West. This expansion of prepaid plans is probably the single most significant change in the underlying organization of medical care in recent decades.

Managed Care, Unmanaged Competition

The original concept of an alternative health-care-delivery system—epitomized by the prototype prepaid group practices, such as Kaiser—has been transformed over the past two decades into the broader and looser concept of "managed care." The first step was the inclusion of IPAs under the HMO rubric; then came the addition of the gatekeeper plans. A still looser alternative, preferred provider insurance (PPI), gives subscribers more complete coverage when they use approved providers who have agreed to accept the plan's rates. While exercising some selective control over providers, PPI plans differ from HMOs in that they provide partial out-of-plan coverage for their enrollees. Even fee-for-service insurance plans with utilization review are now described (to my regret) as managed care. Managed care thus no longer refers only to capitation payment plans but also embraces—at least in the emerging conventional usage—any health plan that limits the choice of providers or regulates their treatment decisions to eliminate inappropriate care and reduce costs (see chart, next page).

Given this diversity of organization, it is not possible to generalize about the overall record of managed care. Prepaid group practices—the organizations for which genuine savings and high quality have been most convincingly demonstrated—now represent only a minority of enrollment in managed-care plans. Many of the newer plans seem to achieve savings, if they do at all, solely by getting discounts from providers (who may then shift costs elsewhere), by denying approval for care or for payment (even though, at least according to subscriber complaints, the care may have been needed), and by enrolling healthier people.

The purpose of broadening the concept of prepaid group practice into managed care was to create a greater variety of health plans, suitable to a great diversity of circumstances and preferences. But, in the process, the image of managed care has become confused and perhaps even poisoned. Many consumers and doctors now associate the concept with a form of remote control—a nurse or bureaucrat at the end of a telephone line refusing approval for a service. Many health-care executives as well as doctors identify managed care with a form of high-pressure sales organization demanding discounts—personified, as one hospital manager once

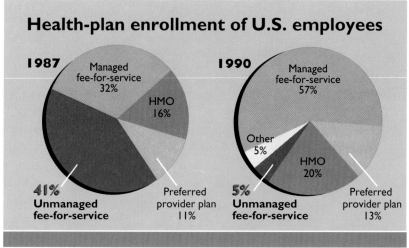

Health-plan enrollment of U.S. employees

1987
Managed fee-for-service 32%
HMO 16%
41% **Unmanaged fee-for-service**
Preferred provider plan 11%

1990
Managed fee-for-service 57%
Other 5%
HMO 20%
5% **Unmanaged fee-for-service**
Preferred provider plan 13%

SOURCES: *HEALTH AFFAIRS*, WINTER 1991; U.S. CONGRESSIONAL BUDGET OFFICE

Although the percentage of employed Americans covered by all forms of managed care has grown sharply, the largest growth has been in plans that rely on traditional payment arrangements.

told me, by the M.B.A. with 10,000 patients in his briefcase who expects, and gets, lower rates.

To be sure, HMOs and other alternatives were bound to create some unhappiness on the part of health-care providers, but they were also supposed to generate savings for employers and, ultimately, consumers. Yet the multiple-choice arrangements introduced by many companies to allow their employees to choose between one or more managed-care plans and conventional insurance have often failed to bring the anticipated savings.

The dynamic at work here was, in fact, quite predictable: under multiple choice, older and less healthy employees—the ones for whom HMOs might achieve the greatest economies in care—tend to remain in the more traditional, fee-for-service insurance plans. As the costs of these options rise, the managed-care plans are able to shadow-price (that is, to raise their rates right behind the price leaders), using the additional revenue to provide better benefits as well as higher profits. As a result, the total cost of all plans may be even higher than it would be if the employer offered conventional insurance alone. In addition, many employers still pay the entire premium for all options, effectively removing any cost-consciousness from consumer choices.

The problem here is not with the original concept of prepaid health care, but with some of the variations on the idea and the inability of employers to counteract the strategies of health plans aimed at escaping responsibility for high-cost patients. It is hard for a health plan to produce high-quality care at a lower price; it is much easier to cut costs by attracting healthy subscribers and getting discounts from providers. Unmanaged competition, therefore, generates a lot of cream-skimming and discounting, which can be highly profitable for the managed-care plan without doing anything to solve the overall problem of health-care inflation.

The apparent failure of the competitive approach to containing health costs is, in a sense, not so different from the apparent failure of the regulatory approach. Halfway reform often does not even reach halfway. The critics of each approach have been quick to leap upon the initial evidence to pronounce the very principles of regulatory limitation and competitive markets at fault. In the early 1980s, some said regulation had been proved ineffective; 10 years later, others said the verdict on competition was the same. But recent experience admits of another interpretation. The regulatory approach failed because it fell short of setting comprehensive budgetary limits, did not control investment, and failed to change incentives. The competitive approach failed because the typical framework established by employers created incentives for opportunism instead of better performance. If we are to get regulatory or competitive strategies right, we have to understand clearly the logic on which they rest.

CHAPTER FOUR

THE LOGIC OF SYSTEMIC REFORM

N othing about health-care reform is more fixed in the public mind than the idea that any improvement will be costly. To be sure, reforms that simply add insurance coverage without altering the financing system would raise spending. But that is not necessarily true of structural reforms that would provide greater financial control over health care, especially compared with a truly expensive policy: doing nothing.

Currently, the annual rate of increase in health costs is more than 10 percent a year on a base of over $800 billion. Each year's growth now far exceeds the one-time incremental cost of covering the uninsured under national health insurance. In fact, according to a 1991 analysis by the Congressional Budget Office, the economies generated by a single-payer system modeled after Medicare would offset the entire cost of additional coverage, producing no net increase in national health costs. A 1991 study by the U.S. General Accounting Office estimated that if the U.S. could reduce its administrative costs to the level in the Canadian system, the savings would actually exceed the cost of covering the uninsured.

Although analysts disagree about how much might be saved in administrative costs, international comparisons and detailed studies of health-care practices suggest that the potential economies to be found in the U.S. system—clinical as well as administrative—are enormous. The challenge of health reform is not to persuade the public to give up beneficial care but to reduce the costs that have no benefit, thereby freeing up the resources needed to include the uninsured within a mainstream standard of health coverage.

Ultimately, this means not just changes in health policy, but an internal transformation in health care. The true objective of systemic reform is to reach deep inside the process of health care and alter the way everyone concerned—doctors, patients, managers—thinks about the decisions they face. At the core of the process are the practice styles of physicians shaping their everyday choices about when to order tests, hospitalization, surgery, prescriptions, and further visits. Reform works best when it promotes a high-quality but conservative practice style—conservative in the sense of conserving resources by proceeding with treatment only when clearly effective. And it is most likely to succeed when doctors, managers, and other health-care professionals work together with patients to arrive at judgments about care through a cooperative rather than antagonistic process.

But how can a more conservative practice style and, I might add, a more conservative style of health-care management be achieved? A changed orientation will not spring up naturally, certainly not under the present system, which has richly rewarded the opposite practices. Nor will it suffice to create public or private regulatory mechanisms that focus on the exceptional cases of gross inefficiency. The crux of the problem is accepted, everyday decision-making.

Two approaches offer what I believe to be the best chance of inducing a shift toward conservative health-care practices and a slowdown in spending. One approach calls for budgetary control from the center; the other for competitive organizations generating decentralized cost-sensitivity. Much has been written about each, often exaggerating the contrast between them. In fact, the two approaches have certain similarities; where they differ, they help remedy their respective weaknesses. A coherent strategy for health reform needs to draw on both.

The Logic of Global Budgeting

To control rising health costs, most major Western countries have eventually found their way to one device: global budgeting, that is, an annually negotiated cap on total expenditures. A global budget may apply to a region, a population, a group of providers, a particular hospital, or (as I shall suggest later) to a private health plan responsible for the comprehensive care of its members. Global budgeting is consistent with a wide variety of ways of organizing health care; it does not necessarily imply a government takeover of health-care finance—in the German system, for example, negotiations among nongovernmental groups set the caps. But it does require enforceable rules about expenditure limits.

Global budgeting also does not mean centralizing detailed budget decisions; rather, it calls only for setting budget ceilings. Ultimately, such ceilings can result in less government regulation than we have today. Once government, employers, and the public are assured that total health-care expenditures will stay within some predetermined limit, they are less likely to pursue the kind of microregulation of health care that the United States has adopted over the past two decades. Global budgeting, therefore, can be more consistent with both the public interest in controlling costs and the professional interest in maintaining clinical freedom. To borrow a metaphor from two physicians who advocate national health insurance, Kevin Grumbach and Thomas Bodenheimer, microregulation is like tying a leash to every cow in a pasture, while global budgeting is like building a fence. Good fences make leashes unnecessary.

Global budgets create a source of countervailing pressure against the health sector's internal impetus toward expansion. The approach seeks to impose a "hard" budget constraint on providers (or the organizations that pay them) to force them to live within limits. The intent is to produce not just fiscal control but new decision-making environments, where health-care professionals and managers come to accept the need to adopt more conservative practices to match available resources to needs.

Thus the aim is to change not just the economics but also the psychology of health-care decisions. The current reimbursement system sets no clear limits; for providers, the object of the reimbursement game is to milk the different sources of payment and, when one resists, to shift costs elsewhere. A comprehensive global budget, however, precludes manipulation of the reimbursement system and encourages managers and physicians to concentrate instead on making the best use of available resources. Instead of promoting an aggressive therapeutic style and an emphasis on high-cost procedures, global budgets encourage less resource-intensive practices that enable providers to manage under constraint. Facing budget limits, doctors and managers are likely to internalize the constraints, gradually altering their rules of thumb about when surgery is really needed or when an expensive new technology genuinely justifies the investment. America's traditional payment system has nurtured therapeutic activism ("when in doubt, take it out"); budget limits nurture therapeutic skepticism ("let's wait and see how this develops"). Given the abundant evidence of excessive surgery, overprescribing, and unnecessary hospitalization, a strong dose of skepticism seems overdue.

Global budgeting for hospitals and for physicians in independent practice has typically involved two different approaches. A global budget for a hospital means a prospectively set, lump-sum payment, instead of reimbursement for itemized services (DRGs are a step in that direction). On the other hand, global budgeting for private physicians might mean (as it has in Germany) annual negotiations between payers and doctors to predetermine a total compensation pool. Physicians would bill into the pool under a relative-value scale and be paid fee-for-service, with fees being adjusted in midyear corrections to keep overall payments in line with the budget. (This is similar to an IPA.) Doctors who overbill do not threaten the insurance funds or the public treasury; they take money away from their peers. Consequently, the government can let the profession decide for itself how to handle such problems.

Global budgeting should be sharply distinguished from price regulation. Price regulation does not guarantee control of total costs because it allows providers to increase the volume of services or shift the mix toward services that are more complex and higher in cost. Nor is global budgeting the same as an expenditure target; if the budget constraint is not hard, it is not a real constraint and will not bring about changes in practice patterns.

Global budgeting should also be distinguished from the rationing of medical care, if that is understood as a scheme for limiting beneficial care according to a scale of priorities, as Oregon has proposed for part of its Medicaid program. The Oregon approach would rank procedures according to likely benefit, cutting off payment for those below a line dictated by available funds. Because of the crude nature of the Oregon ranking—for example, it fails to take a patient's prognosis into account—the system would sometimes deny care to patients with a chance of recovery and approve it for others who have none. By regulating specific clinical situations, Oregon's plan calls for a highly intrusive level of state control. Global budgeting may require tough choices, but it leaves such decisions outside the state to the changing judgments and negotiations of health-plan managers, doctors, and patients. This approach avoids the rigidity of detailed official rules that are likely to become outdated when new scientific discoveries occur.

Critics of global budgeting often liken it to "command and control" central planning. But, on closer inspection, it involves a great deal of decentralization. It is true, however, that as global budget-

ing is usually carried out, it involves regulation of capital investment and planning of health facilities to prevent duplication and
keep the long-range growth of expenditures in check. The disadvantage of such investment controls is that they may block competition and lock outdated patterns of health care in place; and when
the planning forecasts are wrong, shortages may result.

There are two other serious objections to global budgeting. On
its own, global budgeting does not ensure that cost control is
achieved through improved efficiency rather than reduced services
and lengthened waiting lines. Improved efficiency depends on
building into the system rewards for better performance and penal-
ties for worse.

Perhaps more serious, the costs of health care in the United States
are already on a sharp upward trajectory, partly because of policies
that expanded physician training, hospital construction, and medical research. Seventy percent of American doctors are specialists;
countries with successful global budgeting typically have half their
doctors in primary care. While we may try to impose a global budget, the powerful expansionary pressures already at work in the
American health-care system may just bust the lid off. That prospect
suggests we need some other force, working from below, generating other changes to make the system more efficient, innovative,
and responsive to consumer choice.

The Logic of Managed Competition

Managed competition, the design for reform introduced in 1977
by economist Alain Enthoven of Stanford, is one of several models
for using market forces to control health costs and improve the system's performance. The basic idea is to get groups of providers to
compete with each other in a framework that allows consumers to
choose intelligently among them and that encourages cost-con-
scious decision-making. Unlike some other market approaches,
managed competition does not depend for its success on the implausible possibility that consumers will shop around for care when
they are sick, nor does it call for higher deductibles and copayments
as a way of creating greater patient sensitivity to costs. In this approach, the key decision point is the annual choice of a health plan,
a choice made at a time when consumers are not under the pressure of illness and can evaluate alternative plans at different prices.
Under managed competition, these alternatives would consist most-
ly of HMOs and other managed-care plans, as well as one conventional insurance plan offering free choice of provider as long as

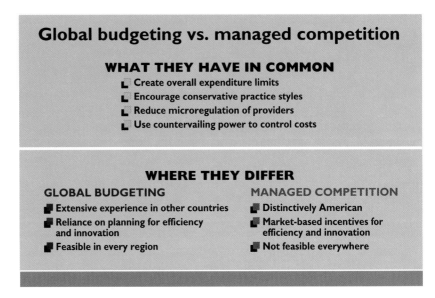

Global budgeting vs. managed competition

WHAT THEY HAVE IN COMMON
- Create overall expenditure limits
- Encourage conservative practice styles
- Reduce microregulation of providers
- Use countervailing power to control costs

WHERE THEY DIFFER

GLOBAL BUDGETING	MANAGED COMPETITION
Extensive experience in other countries	Distinctively American
Reliance on planning for efficiency and innovation	Market-based incentives for efficiency and innovation
Feasible in every region	Not feasible everywhere

that option is able to survive in a competitive framework.

For consumers to make informed choices among these alternatives, the choices need to be presented clearly, with prices that reflect true differences in the plans, not in their enrollees. This is the job of the "sponsor." (Under the current system, the sponsor is usually an employer or a government agency.) The sponsor negotiates the benefit packages, conducts the annual enrollment, provides information to consumers, and collects and disburses payments to plans. Ideally, the sponsor is not merely passive but rather "manages" the competition—hence the name.

Health-plan competition has to be managed because it is susceptible to several predictable problems. First, consumers may have difficulty making informed choices among health plans, especially if there are complex variations in benefits, cost-sharing, exclusions, and so on. Second, health plans can reduce their costs most easily by avoiding high-risk subscribers; thus they have an incentive to discriminate against the chronically ill and disabled and any group believed to be high-risk. To gain a more favorable "risk selection," the plans may even refuse to provide benefits or special services that attract such high-cost groups as alcoholics, HIV-infected individuals, and the mentally ill. Thus, without regulation, a competitive market may well drive out services for the very people who need health care the most.

The ground rules of managed competition are designed to overcome these problems: First, the approach calls for standardized benefit packages among competing plans to enable consumers to make easy price comparisons and prevent the plans from shaping the benefit packages to attract low-risk subscribers. Second, the sponsors would pay the plans according to the risk of the populations they enrolled, thus reducing the incentive to skim off the healthiest and avoid the sick. This practice is known as "risk rating." Finally, the sponsor would have discretionary authority to counteract any opportunistic behavior by plans attempting to enroll only the healthy or to disenroll high-cost subscribers.

These policies are crucial both to control costs and to avoid the inequity—and irrationality—of a health-care system that avoids sick people. One reason for the failure of current multiple-choice plans set up by employers, as I suggested earlier, is that employers have not been able to structure the competition appropriately. When the prices of alternative plans reflect the risk of those who enroll, the price system does not send the right signals. Instead of attracting consumers to the most efficient providers, competition attracts consumers to the healthiest risk pools. The winning plan may well be inefficient in providing health care but clever at marketing.

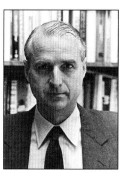

Stanford economist Alain Enthoven introduced the concept of managed competition in 1977.

Thus while managed competition draws on the strengths of a market system, it may also suffer from its potential failures. Competition is not a magic bullet that does away with health-care regulation. In fact, it requires highly skillful regulation by the sponsor. In this respect, it is no different from global budgeting.

Like global budgeting, managed competition moves health care into a world of expenditure limits. Indeed, capitation payment produces a more global budget than do the Canadian and German health-insurance systems, since a health plan paid by capitation works under a comprehensive budget constraint, not just a budget cap on hospital care or physicians' services separately. This is actually a source of greater flexibility; capitation enables health plans to reallocate resources from inpatient to ambulatory services in line with changing preferences and new technology and to introduce nontraditional providers, such as nurse practitioners, in lieu of physicians.

Like global budgeting, managed competition also seeks to generate greater countervailing power to limit provider-induced demand and to create reformed decision-making environments where managers and peers have the incentive and leverage to induce use of more conservative practices. In this model, the impetus comes not only from a hard budget constraint, but also from the threat of competition, which pushes HMOs and other managed-care plans to match their resources to the needs of their members.

The merits of managed competition depend on the kinds of health plans that would grow under the system. As I have suggested, HMOs today include many of the best health-care organizations in the country. They have shown that it is indeed possible to provide high-quality care at significantly lower cost. But not all managed-care plans today exhibit those virtues, and unfortunately, the dominant HMOs in some parts of the country are not admirable organizations. When HMOs are based on multispecialty group practices, they are most likely to pursue lower costs and higher quality by enlisting the cooperation of their physicians in developing conservative practice patterns. But when HMOs are based on doctors in independent, fee-for-service practice, the health plans are much more likely to keep costs under control by pressuring doctors to discount their fees and by requiring telephone approval of hospitalization and other procedures. The result is more likely to be an adversary relationship in which physicians—and their patients— feel they are subject to control by a remote bureaucracy.

Thus the success of managed competition in a region will be greatly affected by its patterns of medical practice. Managed competition seems far more likely to work in the cities and suburbs of the West, where group practice is more common, than in the older metropolitan areas of the East, where solo fee-for-service practice still prevails. Managed competition also faces limits in rural areas throughout the country, where it is often difficult to find a single health-care provider, much less competing alternatives. As a result, managed competition is not an approach that can instantly be used everywhere.

Combining the Approaches

Most analysts of health policy assume that the two approaches I have described lead in opposite directions—global budgeting toward a single-payer system of national health insurance, and managed competition toward a private-sector model. But to pose such a stark choice is misleading.

Any single-payer plan in the United States would have to provide for capitation payment to HMOs and other managed-care plans. If there is capitation, there is the prospect of competition. Competition raises the problem of risk selection and the need to counteract any opportunistic tendency of plans to skim off the healthy and avoid the sick. Consequently, even single-payer plans would have to figure out how to manage health-plan competition.

On the other hand, managed competition does not preclude expenditure limits. As I have suggested, capitation payment is a kind of global budgeting. Consequently, it is entirely possible to have both budget limitation and competition. For example, the Federal Employees Health Benefit Plan, which for decades has provided a choice of HMOs and conventional indemnity plans, has both a budget and a competitive framework. An intelligently designed universal health plan can do the same—indeed, it can do even better.

Thus, despite sharp ideological differences between their advocates, the single-payer model of national health insurance and managed competition are not wholly opposed. To be sure, the single-payer model treats competing HMOs as an incidental feature (and may provide little incentive to use them), whereas the pro-competitive model seeks to assure quality and control of costs by forcing plans to compete by price and service. But even the most ardent advocates of managed competition must recognize that there are geographic and other barriers to carrying out the idea throughout the country. Where managed competition is impractical or where the infrastructure of competitive health plans has yet to develop, global budgeting by a single payer may be the best—albeit second-best—method of containing costs.

The United States faces fundamentally different circumstances today compared with other countries at the time they developed universal coverage. Costs are dramatically higher, and the organization of health care has changed. When Canada and the European countries developed their national health insurance programs, they generally accepted the existing method of fee-for-service payment for physicians. Had the United States adopted national health insurance decades ago, it too would have based its system on fee-for-service medicine. But with the development of HMOs and managed-care plans, the U.S. has now developed a different structure. It would be a mistake, as well as hopeless, to try to turn back the clock, because a plan based on capitation payment and organized systems of care has important advantages.

But the establishment of managed competition and global budgeting and the achievement of universal coverage face a major obstacle: the existing framework of employer-based insurance. If systemic reform means anything, it means transforming that system.

CHAPTER FIVE

BREAKING THE EMPLOYER LINKAGE

Most Americans under age 65 get health coverage through a job—their own or that of some member of their family. Employment is the port of entry, therefore, not only for most consumers but also for healthcare reform. Under the current system, employers determine the kinds of health plans offered to most Americans and the framework of choice. But this raises serious questions: Should Americans' access to health care and the price they pay for it depend on the vagaries of the job market and their employers' benefit policies? Should employers be burdened with managing their employees' health care any more than their housing or education? Are employers the best agents for making these decisions?

Employers began offering health insurance as a fringe benefit a half-century ago, scarcely imagining how much cloth that fringe might ultimately take. The employment-based system has persisted since then due less to a positive belief than to inertia and the difficulty of gaining consensus on an alternative. Today, few on the right or the left defend the employer's role in the provision of health insurance as a matter of principle. Many say that although they would not prefer an employer-based system if we were beginning with a blank slate, it is impractical to change it.

This argument is losing force as well as conviction. Employers do not derive any great benefit from mediating the purchase of health insurance. Many would love to be rid of the burden. As that burden grows, even the most traditional firms are likely to begin asking, Why should we buy our employees health care? Why, indeed.

The Costs of the Employer Linkage

Employment-based health insurance has always had drawbacks, although some have become apparent only with time.

First and most obviously, gaining access to health insurance depends on whether a member of a household is employed and what kind of employment that person has. Part-time and seasonal jobs generally do not qualify for benefits. Children and spouses of employees receive insurance only indirectly, incidentally, and haphazardly. In recent years, the limitations of employment-based coverage of children have become especially severe. Between 1977 and 1987, the proportion of children under age 18 covered by employer-based insurance dropped from 72.8 percent to 62.9 percent. As of mid-1990, more than 25 million children—about 40 percent of all children—lacked employer-based coverage.

Second, the employee group now forms the key risk pool for the spreading of health-insurance costs. Partly because of demographic differences among these groups, some receive relatively low insurance rates, while others face rates that are prohibitively high. Among the losers are those who work for small firms, for companies with relatively older workers, or in occupations believed to create high health risks or to attract workers from high-risk groups.

Third, the system gives employers decision-making power over insurance and medical care. Under traditional insurance plans—those that allow the insured free choice of provider and impose few controls—the employer's power is a relatively minor concern. But the rise of health plans that seek to control costs more aggressively has led employers into micromanaging the health care of employees and their families or selecting agents to do so. This change raises concerns about infringements on liberty and privacy.

Fourth, the tax subsidy of employer-provided insurance is much greater for higher-income than for lower-income Americans. The higher their income, the more likely Americans are to get insurance from their employer, the more generous are those benefits, and the more the tax subsidy is worth. The tax exclusion is a largely invisible federal program that provides subsidies in inverse relation to need: the people with the best insurance coverage get the most federal help to pay for it.

Fifth, employers and the plans they select have shown little ability to control health-care costs. The chief effect of employers' cost-containment efforts has been not to reduce costs but to shift them back to their employees—and sometimes to others with private insurance who have less clout in the marketplace.

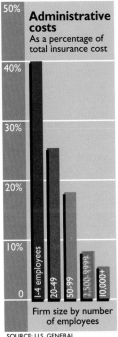

Administrative costs
As a percentage of total insurance cost

50%

40%

30%

20%

10%

0

1-4 employees
20-49
50-99
2,500-9,999
10,000+

Firm size by number of employees

SOURCE: U.S. GENERAL ACCOUNTING OFFICE

Smaller companies may pay as much as 40 percent of insurance premiums for administration, as opposed to actual health services. Large companies may pay less than 10 percent.

Sixth, the employer-based insurance system generates extraordinarily high administrative costs (see chart, left). While Medicare's administrative costs run about 3 percent, private insurers absorb about 13 cents of every premium dollar in marketing and other administrative costs, taxes, and profits—a figure that does not include the administrative costs to the employer, much less to employees and their families. The share of insurance premiums consumed by administration is especially high for medium-size and small employers. For firms with fewer than 50 workers, insurance companies absorb about 25 cents of every premium dollar; for firms with fewer than five workers, insurers take 40 cents.

Seventh, employer-provided insurance has adverse effects on labor-management relations and employment. The system entangles employers in conflicts over health care, drains management time, and leads employers to make increasing use of uninsured part-time and contract workers, who enjoy few rights and little security.

Some may disagree with one or another of the foregoing points. But many conservatives as well as liberals agree that access to insurance ought not to depend on the particular firm one works for, that the tax subsidy is inequitable, and that it is doubtful whether employers acting separately can control costs. The first question of reform, therefore, is whether it is possible to adjust public policies to remedy the many deficiencies of the employment-based system. To answer that question, it helps to understand why employment-based insurance developed in the first place.

Why We Have an Employment-Based System

The linkage of health insurance to employment originally helped to launch and then to broaden insurance protection against the costs of sickness. Until the 1930s, insurance companies did not offer health coverage because the losses appeared impossible to predict. Insurers feared adverse selection (people with high expected costs would be the most likely to take out policies). They foresaw high marketing expenses and collection problems (collecting life-insurance payments then typically required door-to-door agents). And they were concerned that health insurance would not just spread costs but increase them, because the insured would seek more medical care and doctors would raise fees.

This last problem, known as "moral hazard," never was really solved. But the sale of health insurance to employee groups rather than to individuals—pioneered by Blue Cross, which was launched by hospital associations during the Depression—did make private health insurance a workable proposition. Because the employed are a relatively healthy population, group insurance limited adverse selection, and automatic payroll deductions to guarantee payment of premiums cut collection costs. By the late '30s, commercial insurers had entered the market.

When national health insurance plans failed to pass Congress during the New Deal and the Truman years, employment-based health insurance took off, encouraged by World War II-era wage and price controls that exempted employer-paid health-insurance premiums and by federal tax policy that excluded employers' contributions from taxable income. Unions demanded health insurance in collective bargaining, and employers agreed to provide it to attract and keep good workers.

Employment-related insurance grew steadily through the postwar period until the late 1970s. Since then, the percentage of employed Americans who lack health insurance has begun to increase. Manufacturing firms, traditionally generous in their provision of health benefits, have been in decline, while service businesses offering limited or no benefits have expanded. The rollback of health insurance, like the decline of pension coverage, reflects the now indisputable shrinkage of middle-class jobs in the U.S.

The dynamics of the insurance market have also been a factor in declining health coverage. From their beginnings in the 1930s, Blue Cross plans offered health insurance to all employers in a geographic area at the same price, a method known as community rating. Commercial insurance companies, however, provided lower rates to healthier employee groups on the basis of their cost experience (hence the term "experience rating"). This threatened to leave the Blues with the highest-cost subscribers and gradually forced the plans to move away from community rating. In recent decades, insurers have discriminated ever more carefully among groups bearing different risks. This practice, known as market segmentation, inevitably results in the exclusion from coverage of those judged especially high-risk. Today's private insurance system is the outcome of this evolution.

While dozens of proposals to reform the employer-sponsored system are circulating in Congress and in the states, they generally include one or more of four elements: insurance-market reform, mandatory employer benefits, expanded public or publicly subsidized insurance, and tax credits. (Managed competition, another possibility, will be discussed further in the following chapter.) Proposals for incremental reform typically package the components in different combinations in the effort to widen coverage while preserving the role of employers.

Insurance-Market Reform

The purpose of reforming the insurance market is to reverse its recent evolution, re-creating a wider distribution of risk. The leading proposals would prohibit the use of preexisting-condition exclusions (at least in group policies), require the renewal of policies without regard to new illnesses, and either require community rating or limit the range of experience rating in order to reduce prices to groups judged high-risk. Some proposals would also limit annual premium increases. In Washington, Senator Lloyd Bentsen has sponsored legislation for insurance-market reform; under Mario Cuomo's leadership, New York has adopted reforms of this kind.

The political appeal of these measures is clear. They do not require new taxes; instead, they force the insurance industry to reduce prices to high-risk groups and to insure some people now denied coverage. Yet there are some obvious problems.

First, forcing insurers to use community rates and accept all applicants means that while rates may go down for some small firms and high-risk individuals, they will go up for the majority of people who now are insured. Once people feel the effect of the increases, they may conclude that the government has bungled things again. Second, while government can regulate insurance rates, it is more difficult to force private insurance companies to cover high-risk groups they prefer to avoid. Instead, they may adopt ever more subtle risk-avoidance strategies, thereby preventing many people from getting insurance. States that act on their own may also face threats from insurers to withdraw from the market altogether.

Even comprehensive insurance-market reform would still leave millions uninsured. Moreover, it would do nothing to control overall health-care costs or to reduce administrative waste. At most, it would help employees of some small businesses and people with preexisting conditions get more affordable coverage and avoid job lock. But if health costs continue to soar, those who benefit from these reforms will merely face the same problems a bit later.

Insurance-market reform might have its most important effects on the insurance industry itself. Blue Cross and the largest private insurers are big enough to spread risks broadly, and some have invested in the development of managed-care plans. The great majority of smaller insurance companies, however, compete by avoiding risks and rely on techniques that these reforms would prohibit.

Many, perhaps most smaller companies could not survive serious market reform. As a result, such reform might produce a massive consolidation of the health-insurance industry.

Mandating Employer Benefits

One way to extend health coverage is to require all employers to offer it. In the absence of other reforms, however, employer mandates pose serious problems for small and medium-size businesses. For while large employers pay as little as 6 percent of payroll for health insurance, smaller firms pay as much as 12 or 14 percent, or even more. To require firms that do not offer health benefits to suddenly provide them would raise small businesses' costs sharply, lead them to cut back jobs, and perhaps threaten their survival—or so small-business owners fear.

That, however, has not been the experience in Hawaii, the one state that requires all employers to offer health insurance. In 1974, shortly before the enactment of the federal Employee Retirement and Income Security Act (ERISA), which regulates employee benefit plans, Hawaii adopted its health-insurance mandate. Several years later, after a federal court held the mandate in violation of ERISA, Hawaii's representatives persuaded Congress to give the state a special exemption to maintain its system. By most accounts, it has been a success—Hawaii not only has close to universal health insurance, but its health-care costs are no greater than the national average. In some respects, Hawaii is a special case because of its isolation from the mainland and the dominant role in its health care played by two large, competing plans. But the ability of its small employers to pass on the costs of health insurance suggests that small businesses' fear of mandated benefits is exaggerated.

Nonetheless, partly to quiet those fears, proposals for mandatory benefits generally come in combination either with insurance-market reform (to cut down the rates paid for private insurance by small firms) or expanded public insurance available at an affordable price. Under the latter approach, known as play-or-pay, employers would have an option either to play (by buying insurance directly) or to pay a tax for public coverage of their workers. The controlled price of the public program would effectively put a cap on an employer's obligations.

The cost of public insurance to the employer, which would be determined by the payroll tax rate, is the key to understanding the likely effects of play-or-pay proposals. The lower the cost of coverage through the public plan, the more employers will opt for it, thereby creating a larger public program with more middle-class participants. And the more middle-class participants, the greater will be the pressure to maintain adequate standards. A lower public-insurance cost will also cause fewer adjustment problems for firms currently without health-benefit plans. Especially if combined with serious cost controls, such legislation could reduce the burden for employers who currently pay higher rates for insurance.

But it is no longer possible to set a low rate for public coverage without raising additional revenue. Twenty years ago, when health costs were so much lower, public coverage for uninsured working Americans might have cost as little as 4 percent of payroll. Today a payroll tax at that level would not come close to covering employees and their families, much less the unemployed and those outside the labor force. Hence there are two options: a higher payroll tax rate or a second source of revenue (or perhaps both).

The play-or-pay legislation proposed in 1990 by Senator George Mitchell and other leading Democrats includes a formula for determining the cost of public coverage to employers that currently would set the rate at between 8 and 9 percent of payroll. At that rate, there would likely be a large public program enrolling between a third and a half of the population under age 65. Others would be covered by insurance purchased directly by employers.

The difficulties with this approach are fundamental. It would tend to divide Americans into two classes, with the lower tier in the public program likely to have fewer benefits and less financial protection. The structure of play-or-pay, moreover, gives employers, not employees, the power to decide which option to take. Hence many Americans may fear that their employer will "dump" them into a public program akin to Medicaid. In other words, while play-or-pay would be a step up for the millions who have no insurance, it might at least appear to be a step down for the millions who do.

The public program does not have to be like Medicaid. But it would be likely to attract higher-cost individuals and lower-wage groups, which would raise its costs relative to private insurance. In addition, the class makeup of participants in the public program would suggest it was the less desirable option. Voters with employer-provided insurance would have an interest only in containing the costs of the public program, not in improving it; hence political pressure seems likely to be biased in a restrictive direction.

Play-or-pay would also do little to remedy endemic weaknesses in the remaining employment-based insurance system. It would not significantly reduce administrative inefficiencies. It would leave employers in control of health-insurance decisions at a time when health plans are intruding more into patient care. The families of employees changing jobs would often be forced to change health-care plans and providers. When employers and insurers fail, those who depend upon them for coverage would still be left stranded. The inequities of the current system of tax subsidies would remain, although they would not be quite as severe.

Whether or not play-or-pay could control overall health-care costs depends on regulatory measures in the larger legislative package. The Mitchell proposal includes a federal expenditure board that would set annual spending targets and negotiate fee schedules with physicians and other providers to meet the targets—a kind of regulation that is unlikely to control costs because, as I suggested earlier, providers could increase the volume and alter the mix of services. And more regulation may well increase administrative overhead. Although the Mitchell proposal includes various other cost-containment measures such as support for research to improve the effectiveness and efficiency of health-care services, they fail to address the underlying systemic problems. At best, they would be preliminary steps toward more comprehensive reform.

Voluntary Public or Publicly Subsidized Insurance

Yet another route to extend insurance is through direct public subsidies for coverage of the uninsured, without mandating any employer participation. There are several possibilities here:

- Subsidize coverage of high-risk patients by private insurers.
- Allow the uninsured to buy subsidized coverage from Medicaid.
- Set up a separate public insurance plan to provide affordable policies to those who are otherwise uninsured.

The immediate difficulty with all such approaches is their cost. Without employer contributions, the government must raise additional taxes to cover the working poor. Moreover, if employees can get coverage at reasonable rates from a public program without an employer contribution, employers will have an incentive to drop health benefits. As a result, the costs of a public program are likely to grow, perhaps to unmanageable proportions. Such a program would also have high costs because it would cover many people deemed uninsurable by private companies. The combined effect of covering high-risk individuals denied private insurance and inducing employers to drop benefits tends to make such an approach fiscally unsustainable. In addition, many people eligible for public insurance would still decline to pay for it, even at subsidized rates, preferring to take their chances and to use public hospitals if they need care.

Nonetheless, some 24 states have created subsidized high-risk insurance pools; several others, such as Maine and Washington, are subsidizing coverage of the uninsured directly. Typically, these programs do not reach all of the uninsured—in most cases, they reach only a small minority at costs so high that there is no likelihood that they will be extended to cover all the uninsured. Minnesota is the one state to attempt to cover most of the uninsured, but it has a big advantage: the percentage of Minnesotans without insurance is much lower than the national average. Hence the scale of the problem is smaller; even so, the program seems unlikely in practice to cover more than half the state's uninsured.

Tax Credits

The chief element in the conservative remedy for the health-insurance problem is a new program of tax subsidies for the purchase of insurance. In February 1992, President Bush proposed a tax credit of up to $3,750 for families with children ($2,500 for couples and $1,250 for individuals), limited to people with incomes below the poverty line. The proposal also included smaller tax subsidies for health insurance to those above poverty, insurance-market reforms, and provisions to encourage small employers to join health-insurance networks to purchase insurance jointly.

The president's program, however, did not set out any convincing action against the overall growth of health-care costs. (Because of differences within the administration, the proposal also provided no indication of how it was to be financed.) Even if the tax subsidies were fully adopted, millions of Americans—many with incomes above the poverty level—would be left without insurance. Indeed, except for prohibiting preexisting-condition exclusions, the program offered little to relieve insecurity about health insurance among the middle class. And the poor who might acquire insurance with the new tax subsidy would find its value eroding over time because the proposed tax credits are indexed to overall inflation, not to health-care inflation, which is higher.

Moreover, because the program called for the increased purchase of insurance by individuals and small firms, it seemed likely to increase administrative inefficiency. By encouraging small employers to join voluntary networks, the plan hoped to promote greater efficiency in the purchase of insurance. But it is doubtful that such voluntary networks would significantly reduce administrative costs. Indeed, surveys of small employers suggest that the majority would not buy insurance through such networks anyway.

The Limits of Incremental Reform

All the foregoing proposals attempt to build on the foundation of employment-sponsored insurance. This is the strategy of incremental reform. But it is one thing to build on a solid foundation, another to build on a collapsing one. Employment-based insurance is unraveling. There is no sign that employers can control health-care costs. And the more employers do try to control costs, the more they intrude into what ought to be their employees' private decisions about health care. While it is possible in theory to universalize employment-based insurance by providing either tax credits to individuals or a supplementary public-insurance program, these options tend to be extremely costly. They channel more money into a system that shows no ability to control its appetite. And employers do not have the capacity to manage health-plan competition. Paradoxically, it will require public action to create a workable market in health care.

Of the various incremental proposals, play-or-pay offers the best chance of achieving universal coverage and, in principle, could be modified to achieve overall cost control. But it is likely to create sharp inequities in coverage and, therefore, to generate anxiety among those who feel that their insurance may be downgraded. The proponents of play-or-play conceived it as the most politically salable option to achieve universal coverage. But it may be less salable to the public at large than to the corporations and interest groups that have supported the idea. Moreover, it is unlikely to be passed without damaging compromises; and if the support for change is strong enough to avoid such compromises, it would be better mobilized, I believe, on behalf of comprehensive reform.

Compared with incremental reform of employment-based insurance, national health insurance—that is, a system that makes insurance coverage available on the basis of citizenship rather than employment—would provide greater security and economy. But national insurance does not mean that the government has to run the health-care system, or that there cannot be multiple health plans, or that consumers cannot have choice. That depends on the design of reform.

CHAPTER SIX

BUDGET GLOBALLY, CHOOSE LOCALLY

T he previous two chapters have suggested the broad out-lines of a framework for reform: a universal insurance system that provides for consumer choice among competing health plans. It is time to examine more closely how this approach would work.

Fortunately, I am hardly striking out into terra incognita. Many of these ideas have been developed in previous studies, such as those of Alain Enthoven, or in legislation, such as a plan for national health insurance by Senator Bob Kerrey of Nebraska. A similar proposal comes, interestingly enough, from the Catholic Health Association. While related to these models, my approach most closely follows a proposal for California by John Garamendi, the state's insurance commissioner, who drew upon Enthoven's original competition-based national health insurance plan.

The Garamendi proposal, released in February 1992, combines some advantages of a single-payer system with those of managed competition. Instead of acquiring health coverage through employers, consumers would choose a plan through a regional Health Insurance Purchasing Corporation (HIPC). The HIPC, a public authority set up under a state commission, would contract with various HMOs and other managed-care plans as well as one plan offering free choice of provider. These health plans would be owned and run, as they are today, by insurance companies, provider groups, other corporations, or consumer cooperatives. Benefits would be broad and standardized. All plans would have to offer "24-hour" coverage, which would involve merging the health-care components of workers' compensation and auto insurance into a single health-insurance policy, thereby eliminating a lot of duplicate coverage, needless litigation, and excess costs.

Revenue would flow into the HIPC under a payroll tax set at a level sufficient to cover all the state's citizens, except those eligible for federal programs. (Because it was conceived as a measure that California could enact on its own, the Garamendi proposal does not, at least initially, embrace Medicare and Medicaid.) The HIPCs would ensure that at least two plans are available at no additional out-of-pocket premium; other plans might charge more.

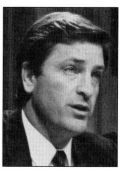

John Garamendi, California's insurance commissioner, whose proposal for reform combines managed competition and global budgeting

This approach would create a single-sponsor system of insurance—the single sponsor being the HIPC, which would assume the functions now performed by employers who arrange for health coverage for their workers. Unlike play-or-pay, the Garamendi proposal does not allow employers to opt out and contract directly for insurance. All revenue for health insurance goes into one pot; the pooling of risk is community-wide. In this respect, the Garamendi approach resembles a single-payer plan: everyone gets health insurance through the same system (although some companies or individuals, using net after-tax income, may choose to buy supplementary policies, say, for uncovered dental care). On the other hand, unlike a single-payer system, Garamendi's single-sponsor approach asks consumers to choose among different health plans at different prices, forcing plans and providers to worry about losing out to more efficient alternatives (see chart, next page). In this respect, the single-sponsor system is market-oriented, pluralistic, and decentralized.

This framework would preserve a role for existing private health plans, but it would greatly change how they compete. Under employer-sponsored insurance, competition among plans easily degenerates into a race to sign up the healthy and avoid the sick. To prevent that, the HIPC would have the necessary staff expertise and authority to manage the competition. Among other measures, it would adjust total payments to health plans according to the risk of their members. It would also monitor disenrollment to ensure that no plan attempted to reduce its costs by inducing high-cost patients to leave. The HIPC would act as the consumer's agent, ensuring fair treatment. And, in a curious twist, the HIPC would be more likely than employers to preserve a free-choice-of-provider option because it would consolidate the current profusion of conventional fee-for-service plans into one plan with a global budget.

The HIPC would not deal directly with doctors or other health-

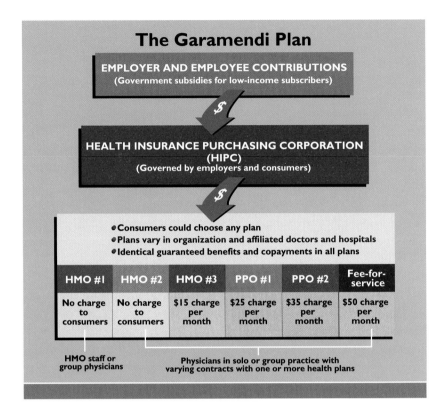

The Garamendi Plan

EMPLOYER AND EMPLOYEE CONTRIBUTIONS
(Government subsidies for low-income subscribers)

HEALTH INSURANCE PURCHASING CORPORATION (HIPC)
(Governed by employers and consumers)

- Consumers could choose any plan
- Plans vary in organization and affiliated doctors and hospitals
- Identical guaranteed benefits and copayments in all plans

HMO #1	HMO #2	HMO #3	PPO #1	PPO #2	Fee-for-service
No charge to consumers	No charge to consumers	$15 charge per month	$25 charge per month	$35 charge per month	$50 charge per month

HMO staff or group physicians

Physicians in solo or group practice with varying contracts with one or more health plans

The dollar amounts cited by Garamendi are for illustration only. They vary because the plans are organized differently and offer different choices of doctors and hospitals.

care practitioners. Rather, it would enable consumers to select one of several privately managed health plans. Doctors and health plans would independently work out the terms of their relationships. To be sure, all the health plans, including the free-choice-of-provider option, would operate under sharper competitive pressures and clearer expenditure limits than now exist outside of HMOs. Undoubtedly, this new framework would affect medical care and the medical profession. Before examining what those effects might be, I want to explore how this model might be financed and developed on a national scale.

Financing and Federalism

Most people approach the issue of finance by sensibly asking, first, how much a program will cost and, second, how we will raise the revenue to pay for it. Unfortunately, much experience teaches that this is backwards. How we pay for health care will determine how much it costs. I exaggerate only slightly.

Imagine that no money were taken from Americans' paychecks and taxes to pay for health care and instead each family received an annual, lump-sum bill for its prorated share of the nation's health expenditures. For 1991, with per capita costs at nearly $2,700, the bill would have been more than $10,000 for a family of four. Under such a system, it is inconceivable that health costs would have been allowed to grow to their present scale.

A key source of high costs in the United States is their fragmentation and obscurity. Reform that proposes to bring them into the clear light of day, therefore, represents a fundamental move toward cost containment. Western countries with national health insurance have lower health costs than the U.S. partly because their expenditures are more visible. To be sure, consolidated financing provides the leverage for cost control, typically through global budgeting. But fiscal arrangements not only raise money; they also help focus opposition. Where health care is wholly financed by general revenues, it has to compete with other national needs such as education and defense and other strong interests that mobilize to keep health spending in check. And where health care is financed by a separate tax, political leaders have to summon the courage and build the support necessary to raise that tax. The difficulty of doing either also tends to retard the growth of health spending.

In the United States, health-care reform not only requires a change in incentives and organization, it requires fiscal clarification as well. Politically, this is just as difficult, if not more so, because the *recognition* of costs is easily confused with an *increase* in costs.

Political instinct favors hiding costs rather than facing up to them. That is partly why insurance-market reforms, mandated employer benefits, and devices such as tax credits and special tax-exempt accounts for health spending are so attractive. They do not seem to cost anything! Yet mechanisms for hiding health costs are exactly what have gotten us into trouble.

If we are to control costs, we are going to have to recognize them, as painful as that may be. Public financing for health insurance should be seen in that context. Those who oppose the approach I am recommending may object that it would—like a single-payer insurance system—require huge tax increases. But the taxes would replace equally huge private-insurance premiums, and from the standpoint of most employees, the deduction of those premiums from their paychecks is already a tax, one whose increases their employers have been unable to control.

Under a plan such as Garamendi's, moreover, the employer and employee contributions would flow directly into a health-care trust fund, which the HIPCs would then disburse to the health plans chosen by consumers. Because the money need not travel to Washington, the public should be less concerned that it will disappear into a black hole inside the Treasury. Their payments for health insurance would pass through a public trust fund, which would pool the risk for the costs of illness in a community, but consumers would determine where the money goes by their choice of plans.

The financing for a single-sponsor system of managed competition need not, however, come from a payroll tax. To keep the financing more like that of the present system, the state could set a flat premium to be paid by employers to the HIPCs on behalf of workers (with fractional payments for part-timers). The employee's share—and the contributions of those outside the labor force with incomes above poverty—could then be collected through the income tax system. To offset the regressive effects of a flat premium, the state (or federal government) could give tax credits to firms with low-wage workers or directly to employees. This approach might be more acceptable politically because the employer contributions to the HIPCs—the bulk of the financing—would be defined as premiums rather than taxes. And the use of tax credits would bring the single-sponsor system closer to models supported by conservatives.

As originally announced, the Garamendi plan would rely on a state payroll tax of 6.75 percent for employers and 1 percent for employees. (Of the total, .75 percent would cover the costs of health coverage now under workers' compensation.) These levies are designed to cover the cost of a standard plan with benefits equal to those of the Kaiser Permanente program—coverage that is more comprehensive than most privately insured Americans enjoy today. It would include physicians' services, inpatient hospital care, laboratory and radiology services, mental health services, some high-cost dental and vision procedures, and outpatient drugs. (There would be no deductibles, but copayments of up to $10 per physician visit and prescription.)

All plans would have to offer the standard benefit package; for a given subscriber population, the HIPC would pay no plan more than it pays the plan (or plans) with the lowest premium. Because consumers who prefer a more costly alternative have to pay for it out of pocket, the public revenue required under this system depends on the most efficient private producers. Under the Garamendi proposal, two clear decisions—one public, the other private—would determine the revenue available for health care: the state legislature's decision about the tax rate that would cover the standard plan, and individual consumers' decisions on whether to buy a more costly option.

Since benefits are the same across plans, one option may cost more than another because it offers different providers, a wider selection of providers, greater convenience, or what consumers perceive to be higher quality—or it may simply be less efficient. In one of its more controversial provisions, the Garamendi proposal places a ceiling on the more costly plans' prices that in California today would limit out-of-pocket premiums to no more than $50 per person per month. Critics object that this cap is unnecessary and would only mean that some affluent consumers would buy more supplementary coverage outside the HIPC instead of within it.

The proposal from Senator Kerrey also calls for a system of universal health insurance that would allow the states to qualify private plans to provide coverage, but it differs from the Garamendi approach in several respects. First, it calls for a state-administered public-insurance plan as the primary insurer; the private plans are alternatives to it. Second, all plans would have to stay within the budget the government provides to them; the Kerrey proposal does not allow the competing plans to charge more to consumers, although it permits them—if they can do so within budget—to add extra benefits to attract enrollees. Third, the plan relies primarily upon national rather than state financing—specifically, a 5 percent payroll tax, plus an increase in the top income tax bracket and various "sin" taxes (cigarettes, alcohol).

Senator Kerrey's approach has some advantages. It is more egalitarian: lower-income beneficiaries would face no price barriers to enrollment in the private options. Some people may feel this feature is more important than the plan's sacrifice of price competition and its probable need for greater revenue (as compared with the Garamendi plan, which requires only enough revenue to pay for the low-cost producer). The Kerrey plan rejects a government insurance monopoly, but it does not seek to use price competition to control costs, relying instead on global budgeting. In effect, Senator Kerrey would say to the health plans: "Go compete with each other by providing the most you can to consumers with this fixed amount of money."

The Catholic Health Association's proposal also calls for federally financed universal coverage with privately organized, globally budgeted health plans ("integrated delivery networks") certified by the states to deliver care. Like the Kerrey proposal, the Catholic plan would rely primarily on a federal payroll tax to fund coverage, but the central insurer would not be state governments. Consumers would choose among private plans, which would compete for enrollment on the basis of their quality and service, not price. The Catholic proposal, like Garamendi's, calls for risk-adjusting payments to plans, and it would set up a state agency to manage the competition among them. However, the association, which represents Catholic hospitals, does not justify its approach in the language of economics; instead, it presents its plan as an expression of Catholic values—an example, perhaps, of the diverse roads different groups may take to arrive at the same policy.

One of the main questions about the Kerrey and Catholic Health Association plans is their forthright reliance on federal taxes. Under any comprehensive proposal, some federal financing will certainly be required, at least if Medicaid and Medicare are integrated into the plan. But it is not clear to me that the federal government should raise all or even most of the revenue for health insurance. Under the Kerrey proposal, the responsibility for controlling costs would lie primarily with the states. Yet because the federal government would provide nearly all the funds, the states might not have a strong enough incentive to be vigilant. To ensure the proper balance of fiscal responsibility, therefore, the states should have to raise much of the revenue, as they would under the Garamendi proposal.

Another reason to rely on the states is the regional diversity of health-care organizations and the difficulty of prescribing a single solution for the entire country. Successful reform will have to involve devolution—that is, moving many decisions about health insurance downward in the federal system. Devolution does not have to compromise the fundamental goals of reform. Even in Canada each province has its own health-insurance system, operating within the framework of national guidelines. In the United States, primary responsibility should also belong to the states.

The federal role in health care can be less extensive than it is today. My view is that the federal government should prescribe broad minimum criteria for acceptable universal insurance programs to be organized by the states and offer part of the financing to help the states carry out the programs. In addition to continuing to pay for Medicare beneficiaries, the federal government would subsidize the inclusion of low-income consumers in a mainstream standard of coverage. As the new system was phased in, the federal government would abolish Medicaid and provide support for universal coverage in fixed per capita contributions, graduated according to income. The funds might go to the states or directly to consumers in the form of vouchers redeemable through the HIPCs. Unlike entitlement programs, the cost to the federal government would not depend on the volume or type of health services used. Under this system, the federal government would have no relation with specific providers; it would not set hospital rates or physician payment policies.

The states might not either. Together, the federal and state governments would determine the revenues available to the HIPCs, which would then contract with various health plans. In effect, this puts the health-care system on global budgets (although, again, it does allow consumers to put in extra money to buy an option more expensive than the low-cost plan). Except for Medicare, which would necessarily have to be phased into the new system over time, the federal government and the states could get completely out of the business of determining reimbursement levels, leaving them to be negotiated privately by the plans and the providers. The federal government would neither regulate the rates of providers nor bar states from doing so; whether to deregulate provider prices is a choice the states should make based on their varied circumstances.

A strong federal regulatory and financial role would still be needed in certain areas such as medical education and research. Physician training raises some special problems. Neither the states nor individual health plans can reduce overspecialization among physicians. The federal government has long subsidized specialty training programs; it is time to reverse that policy, to shut down excessive subspecialty training programs and promote primary care. Unfortunately, even with universal insurance, market forces are also unlikely to bring enough doctors into poor communities. As a result, the federal government will need to maintain the National Health Service Corps, making financial assistance for medical students contingent on commitments for subsequent work in underserved areas. The HIPCs, too, will have to take additional steps to ensure adequate service in poor communities. As a condition for participation, they might require plans in their region to locate clinics in or near poor neighborhoods, or to enroll some minimum number of voucher-subsidized consumers. The HIPCs should also make poverty one of the risk factors in calculating payments to the plans to help interest the plans in serving the poor.

The federal government also has a legitimate role to play in setting standards for health care. The Jackson Hole Group, an independent group of competition-oriented health-care reformers that includes Enthoven and Paul Ellwood, has proposed modeling a new national standard-setting process for health care after the system that sets financial accounting rules. Just as the Securities and Exchange Commission, an independent federal agency, relies on the work of the private Financial Accounting Standards Board, so a new National Health Board would rely on designated private bodies to develop medical practice guidelines and uniform standards for health-care organizations. Federally endorsed medical practice guidelines, while not mandatory, would help provide support for conservative practice patterns both in public opinion and in court, if those patterns were challenged in malpractice suits. (Under Minnesota's recent health-reform legislation, adherence to guidelines developed by the state will constitute a clear and convincing malpractice defense.) Uniformity in the reporting of data about health care would help the public hold health plans accountable for their quality as well as cost. In general, the better the information consumers have about health care, the less government should have to intervene. Here is where a new framework of choice and of countervailing power can help disentangle government from management of the health-care system.

The Organization of Choice

There are two polar theories about "choice" in health care. One theory maintains that patients should have an unrestricted right to choice of *provider*. The second maintains that consumers should have a right to choice of *health plan*. The American Medical Association used to say that any health plan limiting choice of physician violated an essential freedom and should be banned. Many states agreed and as recently as the early 1970s did prohibit such "closed-panel" health plans, now known as HMOs. In contrast, the advocates of competition and defenders of HMOs have charged that the AMA's practices and restrictive laws denied consumers free choice by suppressing alternative organized systems of care.

These different interpretations of choice are still with us. Today, some employers continue to offer a single insurance plan with free choice of providers, while others provide employees a choice of plans, most or all of which restrict the choice of providers. In the design of health-care reform, the same choice about choices arises: Should there be a single health plan with free choice of providers, or multiple plans with limited choice? Or should there be a third possibility—multiple plans, including at least one with free choice of providers?

Advocates of a Canadian-style or single-payer approach call for one universally available insurance plan allowing patients to choose whatever private physician or other provider they want. This, interestingly enough, is the AMA's old fee-for-service model on a universal scale. Some other proposals, hoping to preserve employment-based insurance, might turn all health care into managed care; consumers would choose among plans, none of which would allow free choice. The single-sponsor approach is a compromise. It seeks to create a system composed primarily of competing HMOs and other managed-care capitation plans, but it also aims to preserve a free-choice-of-provider option.

Indeed, the single-sponsor approach has a greater capacity to preserve that option than does an employer-sponsored system. Traditional free-choice options offered by employers are being crushed by adverse selection and by the inability of fee-for-service providers to contain costs. The single-sponsor approach, on the other hand, would use risk-rating and other mechanisms to prevent free-choice options from experiencing higher costs solely because older, sicker subscribers, with long-established relations to doctors, are more likely to enroll in them. In addition, global budgeting promises better control of the total costs of health care outside the HMOs and managed-care plans.

Under the single-sponsor approach, the free-choice-of-provider option would be unlike conventional indemnity insurance today: it would have a fixed budget. In regions where there is little competition, such as rural areas, the principal health plan or the HIPC itself would most likely negotiate global budgets with hospitals. Elsewhere, depending on state policy, global hospital budgets might be set in negotiations under the auspices of the HIPC involving all plans in a region. As in the German system, the total compensation pool for physicians outside managed-care plans would also be fixed annually. Physicians would be paid fee-for-service, but the value of fees would depend on the volume and mix of services and the size of the compensation pool.

The interest in preserving a free-choice option is one reason to restrict the proliferation of insurance plans. The single-sponsor approach would allow only one free-choice option. Without this restriction, control of risk selection, reduction in administrative costs, and global budgeting of fee-for-service physician compensation would be difficult, if not impossible. The single-sponsor approach also bars employers from opting out and contracting directly with insurers for the same reason—to prevent a multiplication of payers from undermining cost containment. If opting out were allowed, the HIPC would be left—like the public plan under play-or-pay— with the less favorable risks, as the healthiest employee groups sought cheaper rates. Such a process tends to feed on itself, leaving behind, as it were, the halt, the lame, and the blind. As a result, the costs of insurance obtained through the HIPC would grow, compromising its ability to offer a comprehensive benefit package.

To be sure, if the system allowed employers to opt out, some healthy employee groups would benefit from not having to pay for community-wide health risks. But why should people who happen to work at large firms enjoy this advantage over those who work at small firms? This is essentially a tax exemption for which there is no good justification. The lost revenue from those groups would make costs higher for everyone else and undermine the credibility of the system as a mechanism of cost-control.

In addition, with millions of people remaining under employment-based insurance, we would have all of the problems that now beset that system: insecurity of coverage, discontinuities whenever people change jobs, and intrusion by employers into employees' private choices about their health care. While a single-sponsor plan denies companies the ability to opt out, it creates a framework in which the employees are likely to have many more choices than a single employer can give them. This is a fair trade-off: the employees of big firms share in community-wide health risks (determined under this approach by the low-cost producer), but they get a wider range of choice, greater security, and freedom to change jobs without disruption of ongoing health care.

The Impact on the Medical Profession

Universal health insurance based on competing private plans would have some clear-cut advantages for doctors over other proposals for reform. This approach would leave physicians with a variety of different practice options, from fee-for-service to staff-model HMOs. The model's pluralism would avoid subjecting physicians to comprehensive all-payer fee regulation. And especially if Medicare can be integrated into this system, there would be much less federal regulation altogether.

But I do not want to pretend that physicians would benefit economically from this model. According to a study by two health economists, Gregory Pope and John Schneider, national spending on physicians' services doubled in real terms between 1980 and 1989, up from $63.1 billion to $117.6 billion in constant 1989 dollars. Over the decade from 1978 to 1988, they estimate that real net income—that is, after expenses and after inflation—rose 46 percent for surgeons, 24 percent for medical specialists, and 9 percent for general and family practitioners. It seems highly unlikely that under the system I am suggesting either total spending on physicians' services would have grown as fast or that surgeons would have benefited as much. Global budgets would have restrained the growth of the pool of funds for physician compensation, and competitive health plans would probably have concentrated a larger share of surgical procedures in fewer hands, intensifying competitive pressures on surgeons to cut fees.

Yet it is unlikely that the plans would have entirely blocked growth in physician spending or spread income gains equally among physician specialties. The surgeons' rising incomes reflected both higher profit margins (which are vulnerable to competitive forces) and an increased volume of complex procedures. Surgeons are benefiting in part from a technological explosion that is unlikely to quiet down anytime soon. HMOs and managed-care plans, moreover, will not be in a position, even under this proposal, to dictate terms to doctors because they will need physicians' cooperation to control overall health costs. Or to put it another way, doctors can save money for health plans, not just by keeping down increases in their own fees but also by conserving health-care resources. And from the health plans' standpoint, the latter may be far more important.

The development of a competitive system is unlikely to threaten the existence of private medical practice. As they do today, health plans will generally find it in their interest to contract with independent physicians and physician groups. Even among prepaid group practices, the group-model plans (where physician groups are independent of the plans) seem to have better growth prospects than do staff-model plans. Indeed, as Alan Hillman and his colleagues at the University of Pennsylvania have pointed out, one of the key features of many HMOs is an intermediate physician organization that exercises the real control over how doctors are paid and regulated. So while the development of a competitive system may push doctors to organize themselves into more multispecialty group practices, recent experience does not suggest the plans will seek to buy out the groups and run them directly.

In areas such as California and Minnesota where there is already intense health-plan competition, the Garamendi proposal and others along the same lines would not dramatically alter the conditions of medical practice. Of course, it is hard to foresee all the consequences of financing reform. But whatever the general trends, many practitioners would find their professional work little changed from what it is today—except that all their patients would have health coverage, under one plan or another.

Providing for Children and the Elderly

Several groups with special needs merit special attention. I cannot deal with all such cases, but I want to suggest at least briefly what allowances ought to be made for two groups—children and the elderly.

The health-care needs of children have never received proper attention in our health-insurance system. "Insurance" is not even the appropriate conceptual framework for children's health services because the problem is not so much to insure against unpredictable risks as to provide for preventive care, health education, and much routine treatment of sickness. A lot of health care for children is also almost indistinguishable from education because it is concerned with managing behavioral problems.

One possibility, under the system I have described, would be to allow families to make separate decisions for adults and children. Today, when employees are offered a choice of health plan, they are asked to make a single choice for the entire family. Under this proposal, families would make two choices. That would encourage health plans to compete for children and thereby promote attention to children's services. Moreover, it would permit the development of capitation plans—perhaps with clinics based in schools—focused on children's health.

Capitation payment makes especially good sense for children's services because it would allow a health plan to orient itself to preventive and behavioral services that are not reimbursable under typical insurance arrangements. And separating children's enrollment from that of adults would allow parents who prefer a more conventional insurance arrangement for themselves to sign their children up with a health maintenance organization or school-based children's health service oriented more to preventive and behavioral concerns. Such an approach would be more beneficial to children—and, ultimately, to the adults they become—than merely providing coverage of high-tech medical intervention.

If only because of Medicare, the system will also have to provide separate treatment for those over 65. Like children, the elderly ought to have some special options. Those now on Medicare should have the right to remain in a traditional free-choice-of-provider arrangement. However, the federal government should begin converting the structure of Medicare to a choice model by conducting an annual enrollment with new managed-care alternatives (which might include Medigap and even long-term-care coverage in a single package). The ultimate goal should be to put Medicare on the same footing as the rest of the system, where coverage is comprehensive and costs are globally budgeted, determined by the low-cost producer, and held down by competitive forces and more conservative treatment norms. But it may be easier to make this change for new Medicare beneficiaries than for the elderly today. From the federal government's standpoint, Medicare is a "defined benefit" obligation, while the system I am describing is a "defined contribution" system. That is, under Medicare, the federal government is obliged to pay whatever it costs to provide the services to which beneficiaries are entitled. Under the approach proposed here, the federal government's obligation would be for a specific monetary contribution. In the long run, this change is essential to control federal health costs, but it is politically unrealistic to think that Medicare could be wholly converted tomorrow.

Much more will have to be done to control the health-care costs of the elderly. More than for any other age group, changes in practice patterns and cultural expectations are necessary to limit expenditures that do little but prolong dying. The reform of health care for the elderly should also be intertwined with the revival of nonmarket social ties through such measures as time banks, which enable the well elderly to help the sick and thereby accumulate rights to help from others in turn. Ultimately, there will be no choice but to make long-term care part of Social Security. However, our ability to undertake that task will be much greater if we have more comprehensive health-care systems that can serve as gatekeepers to long-term-care institutions and prevent costs from escalating uncontrollably.

FROM HERE TO REFORM

Reformers have been waiting for the Big Bang in health insurance for more than 75 years. Several times universal health insurance has seemed almost within reach, only to recede as opposing interests mobilized and windows of political opportunity closed amid wars and recessions. Perhaps a similar scenario will unfold in the 1990s. The trend of the past decade has been for Americans to lose health coverage, not to gain it. As costs rise, more employers may drop benefits, new businesses may start without any, and public programs may be cut. The negative consensus on health care could simply grow more negative without any positive consensus taking shape.

Yet, with perhaps typically American optimism, I do not really believe that will happen. To be sure, many people prefer the status quo to change. But the status quo is itself changing, as rising costs threaten interests great and small. All the trends suggest that the need for reform will increase, until finally the barriers break. At that point, I believe it will become apparent to the major interest groups in health care that they will not be able to get their preferred choices for reform.

Twenty years ago, it was possible to conceive of a national health insurance program with no controls on providers. Such was the original framework of Medicare. That approach is no longer plausible, however, as the subsequent history and growing financial burden of Medicare itself indicate. To ensure economic security to individuals, national health reform must include universal coverage. To provide economic security to the country, it must now simultaneously be a program for cost containment.

Today the organizations representing physicians, hospitals, and other providers do not object to universal coverage if it comes without financial controls. That would increase the flow of revenue into health care without restricting their autonomy. Insurers do not object to universal coverage as long as it is achieved by injecting more money into the existing insurance system, for example, through tax credits for purchasing private policies. Consumers, too, would like to have it all: comprehensive coverage, no out-of-pocket costs, no restrictions on choice, and, of course, no tax increase either!

If these illusions are the standards for judging acceptable reform, we are more likely to have universal disappointment than universal health coverage. Ultimately, the well-organized interests in health care will have to ask themselves which second-best alternative they are prepared to accept. Employers must ask if they want to manage their employees' health care. And consumers, who ultimately bear the costs, must ask themselves which approach offers the best value for their money.

Why Good Policy May Make a Good Compromise

I have outlined an approach to reform that emphasizes a few core concepts: national—that is, citizenship-based—health insurance, global budgets, managed competition, and the disentanglement of both employers and the federal government from management of the health-care system. I have argued for this approach on its merits, not its political appeal. It may not be any interest group's first choice, but I believe many groups will find it an acceptable compromise.

Ideologically, this is a hybrid—a form of universal social insurance that deemphasizes the federal role and calls for greater price competition. No doubt some on each end of the spectrum will consider it heresy, and others will simply find it puzzling. It certainly will not fit on a bumper sticker. But it has a coherent logic, and, although it corresponds to no other nation's system, it reflects the experience of other countries and of successful health-care organizations in the United States.

To consumers, this approach offers security, access, and choice. No one would need to worry about losing health coverage after losing or changing a job, about being forced to find a new doctor because of a change of employer, or about a sudden termination of benefits by an employer with a self-funded benefit plan. All would enjoy a broad, mainstream standard of coverage and have the right to choose among different health plans competing for their favor in a system that offered strong consumer protections.

This approach guarantees the poor a ticket of admission to the health-care system. By no means would it solve all their health problems—many of those are inextricably interwoven with other social conditions—but it would be a major step toward social inclusion. For the middle class, it would provide financial protection without disrupting existing health-care arrangements. Through the HIPCs they will be able to secure the coverage their employers now offer. Some in the middle class may face stronger incentives to enroll in HMOs and managed-care plans; millions of others will gain new alternatives their employers could not make available.

The healthy affluent may have to pay more for coverage, although if the authors of legislation are prudent, they will resist the temptation to use health-insurance legislation to solve the problems of income distribution. (If troubled by that thought, they should look up Franklin D. Roosevelt's defense of the decision to finance Social Security by a payroll tax in 1935 and reflect on the collapse of the Medicare catastrophic care plan when the affluent elderly revolted immediately after its adoption in 1988 because of its progressive financing.) For the affluent who want to buy extra coverage or what they believe to be the best care, this approach poses no obstacles. It seeks to include the poor in a mainstream standard of coverage and to assure the middle class of security, not to restrict the rich. It seeks to eliminate inequalities at the bottom, not at the top.

Providers should be able to live with this approach, too. It offers overall stability for the industry, maintenance of private entrepreneurship, and significant federal deregulation. There are firm budget constraints, but there is the prospect of less microregulation.

The biggest changes will affect the health-insurance industry. This approach does not exclude insurance firms from the market, but it does require that they transform their role. To those health-insurance companies that have invested in managed care or that are prepared to run the consolidated free-choice options under the HIPCs, this alternative offers major opportunities.

Undeniably, many small health-insurance companies, various brokers, and other intermediaries will have to look for new businesses or new jobs. To reduce the excessive administrative costs in our system, reform of almost any sort will have to bring about a consolidation of the insurance industry. Because administrative costs for private insurance run as high as 40 cents on the premium dollar for the smallest employers, this is one place where the surgeons of health policy have no choice but to operate.

Yet the health-care system is scarcely going to shrink; the objective is to contain its growth. Even if the health-care sector could be held at 13 percent of GNP, which seems improbable, this proposal will provide plenty of income to go around for those who provide health care, organize it, or invest in it.

A narrow defense of economic interests will be self-defeating for the medical profession and other provider groups. The era of limits has been long in coming; its arrival has been delayed, but it is certain. Rather than struggling to maintain the status quo, physicians would be much better served by taking a positive role in bringing about change, as many have done in recent years. The medical profession has legitimate interests that ought to be addressed in any overall compromise reform package. Earlier I suggested that malpractice litigation is not a major reason for higher health costs. But physicians have a reasonable concern about malpractice suits threatening their economic security. If health-insurance reform can assure security to the public, surely we can find some way to assure security to physicians without compromising quality assurance.

Perhaps the most strenuous opposition to this proposal, as to any universal-insurance plan, will come from small businesses that now do not pay anything for employee health benefits. They will claim that the new payroll taxes will cost jobs and jeopardize their survival. If these taxes were to fall on them exclusively but not their competitors, they would have more of a case. But it is precisely because health costs are now distributed so unevenly among businesses that their case is so weak. Many small businesses that avoid paying for health insurance are taking a free ride, letting others pick up the cost of their employees' unpaid hospital bills. Moreover, the evidence suggests that higher employer contributions for health insurance, whether as premiums or payroll taxes, come out of wages or are passed along in higher prices. (Recall, however, that such costs are higher in the United States than in other countries precisely because we have no comprehensive system for financing—and controlling—costs.) Small employers survived handily in Hawaii after health benefits were required by the state; recent studies of federal increases in the minimum wage show little adverse effect. Small-business proprietors envision worse effects from a tax for health benefits because they are thinking not about the comprehensive effects on labor markets and their competitors or the long-run effect on the health system, but only about the short-run impact, as if their business alone were being asked to pay.

Ironically, a lot of small-business owners and employees suffer from the current system because of the disproportionately high insurance rates they are quoted. Reform would allow them to acquire coverage at a far better price than they can get now. They will also be offered some special concessions; the Garamendi proposal, for example, suggests a lower tax rate for smaller businesses. Of course, for all business the real payoff lies in slowing the rate of increase in health costs. Among other effects, that will reduce the likelihood that other taxes will have to be raised. Good policy is ultimately in everyone's interest.

The Transition to Citizenship-Based Health Insurance

The transition to universal insurance is inevitably complicated because of the health-care system's current hidden and uneven costs and variable benefits. Some people who pay little, or think they pay little, will object because they suddenly see what appear to be (and perhaps are) larger costs. Others will fear that they will lose a special benefit offered by their employer.

Such fears are highly combustible. To prevent them from turning into a political firestorm, Congress would be wise to make some changes in advance of the main body of reform and to build in various transitional measures. As an initial step, employers should be required to declare the full cost of their health-benefit plans in their regular wage and salary reporting to employees as well as the government. Employees must begin to understand how much of their compensation is going to health care, and how rapidly the cost is rising. In some cases, the payroll taxes to be paid under universal insurance will actually be less than employers are now paying in premiums. Employers should be required to return to their employees some portion of the savings—say, 50 percent—in the form of supplementary benefits or a one-time wage increase.

The tax system can help smooth the transition and offset the gains and losses. Small businesses that previously paid no health benefits should receive temporary adjustment assistance through the federal tax system. On the other hand, businesses with large liabilities for retiree health costs will suddenly reap windfall savings from publicly financed health insurance. The federal government should capture a portion of this windfall, which would run in the hundreds of billions of dollars, to help pay for other transitional costs associated with the program.

Cutting the employer linkage is the biggest institutional shift in the approach I am advocating. Following Alain Enthoven's better-known model for a "consumer choice" health plan, many who support managed competition envision fitting it into the employment-based insurance framework, at least for large firms. They advocate mandating all employers to provide health insurance and requiring only small to medium-size businesses to buy insurance through the HIPCs. Because small business could not opt out of the HIPCs, this arrangement does not create as big a risk of adverse selection for the HIPCs as would be faced by voluntary health-insurance purchasing cooperatives, such as those President Bush has proposed.

Yet retaining employment-based coverage for large firms would cause major problems. It would greatly reduce the prospects for effective cost control because the HIPCs would not be able to establish global budgets in a consolidated insurance system. It would leave large employers with the task of managing health-plan competition (insofar as they did offer choice), and there is no sign that employers can do so effectively. It would mean that many employees and their families would face disruptions of care and discontinuities of coverage when the breadwinner changes jobs.

To be sure, this approach would get the HIPCs up and running and make health-insurance coverage universal. If the omission of large firms were planned as a short-term transitional measure, it might allow the HIPCs needed time to gear up to full operation. In structuring the transition, as in other areas, allowance needs to be made for diverse approaches among the states.

National Reform Without a National Bureaucracy

One recent study of public opinion about health care quoted a man from Flint, Michigan, saying, "I am for national health care, but I don't want the government involved." Opponents of national health insurance have seized upon the statement as evidence that the public is confused about rather than strongly supportive of national health insurance. I take the man's position to be entirely reasonable. National health care—yes, in the sense that all citizens must have access to coverage and care. The national government managing health care—no. Even Canada's federal government does not manage the system; in fact, the total number of federal employees concerned with national health insurance in Ottawa is fewer than two dozen.

The approach I have proposed calls for universal health coverage with minimum federal standards, but the organization would be doubly decentralized. It relies upon private health plans to assume the risks of health costs and deliver services and upon the states to establish regional authorities to structure the competition.

But I do not assume that this model will draw universal approval or that it can be carried out equally well throughout the country. The federal government should accommodate various approaches among the states, allowing them to experiment within a framework of minimum criteria for coverage and cost containment on a schedule that would move rapidly to universal insurance.

Currently, many states are experimenting with policies to control costs and expand access, and all are struggling with out-of-control Medicaid budgets. But federal law severely restricts the states' ability to make health policy. The most serious constraint is ERISA, the federal law that bars the states from regulating employee health-benefit plans, even though the states have the authority to regulate health insurance. The courts have interpreted ERISA to mean that state insurance laws apply only when employers buy coverage from insurance companies, not when they self-fund their benefits. As a result, more employers have self-insured, and the states have gradually lost not only effective control of health insurance but any realistic possibility of reforming health-care finance. Today, because of ERISA, state initiatives are seriously handicapped.

Other constraints are also severe. For important Medicaid innovations, the states generally need a federal waiver; Medicare is entirely off-limits. Curiously enough, therefore, national reform requires in some respects that the federal government deregulate the states.

But it must go further than that. In devising universal insurance, the federal government should offer the states a menu of alternatives. In addition to the single-sponsor approach to managed competition that I favor, the federal government should allow mandated benefits, play-or-pay, or a state single-payer plan. Hawaii has a reasonably successful system of mandated employer benefits; Vermont may prefer a single-payer plan; California may go for the Garamendi approach. Providing for diverse solutions not only has political appeal; it is potentially an important source of learning. So, while I am convinced that the approach I have described makes better sense than other alternatives, I recognize that not everyone shares my conviction. We will be better off if the states undertake different strategies of reform, even if some fail, than if the nation as a whole continues to be deadlocked because we cannot agree on one system for all.

I said earlier that national health reform is not like a riddle without an answer. Neither is it like a problem in arithmetic to which there is only one right answer. Around the world are diverse systems of health-care finance that appear to perform better than ours, and at home we have many positive examples of alternative ways of organizing insurance and medical care. It is the task of political leadership to secure an agreement on a design for reform that is at least acceptable to the many who may fail to get their preferred solution adopted. One way to do that is to let some choices devolve onto the states. Public-opinion polls often find majority support for conflicting remedies to the health-care crisis, and some observers suggest, therefore, that the polls mean nothing. A more reasonable interpretation, it seems to me, is that although they do not understand the technicalities, many Americans feel they could probably live with more than one approach. But they want their leaders to act.

Many people today are skeptical that the federal government can act rationally on health insurance or, for that matter, on anything else. Opponents of reform call upon that cynicism to discourage strong, comprehensive action. In a sense, they have laid down a challenge to democratic government: Are we simply destined to let the crisis of health costs and health insurance unfold? Or can we summon the positive agreement on reform that has yet to emerge from the clash of interests and the buzzing, unfocused confusion of our political debate? If representative government in America cannot soon achieve that positive consensus on as urgent a concern as health care, we are truly in trouble.

ADDITIONAL COPIES

To order copies of *The Logic of Health-Care Reform* for friends or colleagues, please write to The Grand Rounds Press, Whittle Books, 333 Main St., Knoxville, Tenn. 37902. Please include the recipient's name, mailing address, and, where applicable, primary specialty and ME number.

For a single copy, please enclose a check for $21.95 plus $1.50 for postage and handling, payable to The Grand Rounds Press. Quantities may be limited. Discounts apply to bulk orders when available. For more information about The Grand Rounds Press, please call 800-765-5889.

Also available, at the same price, are copies of the previous books from The Grand Rounds Press:

The Doctor Watchers by Spencer Vibbert
The New Genetics by Leon Jaroff
Surgeon Koop by Gregg Easterbrook
Inside Medical Washington by James H. Sammons, M.D.
Medicine For Sale by Richard Currey
The Doctor Dilemma by Gerald R. Weissmann, M.D.
Taking Care of Your Own by Perri Klass, M.D.

Please allow four weeks for delivery.
Tennessee residents must add $8^{1}/_{4}$ percent sales tax.